JULIUS WAGNER-JAUREGG

The financial support of Glaxo in the publication of this book is most gratefully acknowledged by the Publisher.

Julius Wagner-Jauregg (1857–1940)

Magda Whitrow

To Michael
with every good
wish and heavy
thanks for making
me laugh
Magda

SMITH-GORDON
NISHIMURA

Smith-Gordon and Company Limited
Number 1, 16 Gunter Grove, London SW10 OUJ, UK
Tel: +44 71 351 7042   Fax: +44 71 351 1250

Nishimura Company Limited
1-754-39 Asahimachi-Dori, Niigata-Shi 951, Japan
Tel: +81 252 23 2388   Fax: +81 252 24 7165

© 1993, Magda Whitrow
Publishing Manager: Joanne Murray
Publisher: Eldred Smith-Gordon

British Library Cataloguing in Publication Data

A catalogue record for this book is available from the British Library

ISBN: 1-85463-012-1

Typeset by Best-Set Typesetter Ltd, Hong Kong.
Printed and bound in Great Britain by
Whitstable Litho Printers Ltd, Whitstable, Kent.

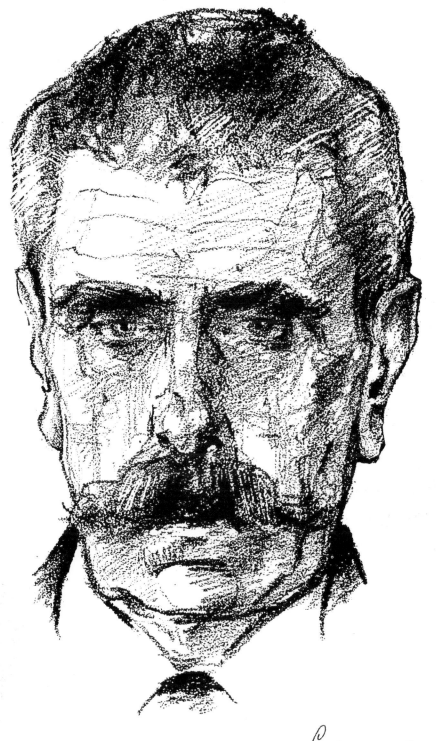

Ich beabsichtige einen Teil der mir noch beschiedenen Lebenszeit dazu zu verwenden, um Erinnerungen aus meinem Lebenslauf aufzuzeichnen. Ich tue das zum Teil, um mein Gehirn zu entlasten. Ich bin nicht im Stande untätig zu sein. Nichtige Zerstreuungen, wie z. B. Kartenspielen, ev. Schachspielen, in Gesellschaft schwätzen und Geschwätz anhören, interessiren mich doch nur ganz vorübergehend. Wenn ich mich aber mit wissenschaftlichen Arbeiten zu lange beschäftige, wird mir der Kopf voll und es fühle mich nicht wohl. Aber das blosse zwanglose Niederschreiben von Erinnerungen dürfte mich vielleicht nicht anstrengen sondern eher entspannen.

Ich weiss zwar nicht, ob diese Blätter nach meinem Tode noch viele Menschen interessiren werden. Von meinem Sohne nehme ich das zwar an. Ob das bei meinen Enkelkindern, wenn sie einmal das entsprechende Alter erreicht haben werden, noch der Fall sein wird, bezweifle ich. Bleibt noch meine Frau und Tochter Julie sowie die Familie Ungethüm.

Vielleicht wird dann auch noch einer oder der andere meiner älteren Collegen vorhanden sein, der sich für das eine oder andere Capitel interessirt.

Ich wünsche nicht, dass diese Erinnerungen oder Teile derselben gedruckt werden sollen. Am wenigsten soll etwas davon in die Hände der Journalisten fallen. Ueber die habe ich mich mein ganzes Leben hindurch genug ärgern müssen. Jeder Stand hat seine Vorzüge und seine Fehler. Ich glaube bei den Journalisten überwiegen die Fehler ungemein, wenigstens bei der Mehrzahl der Individuen die jetzt dieser Gilde angehört. Vielleicht wird das einmal anders, wenn das „Internationa" aus der Journalistik verschwindet.

I intend to devote part of the time still granted to me to record some reminiscences of my life. I am doing this partly to take the pressure off my brain. I cannot be idle. Vain diversions, such as playing cards or chess, talking to others or listening to their chatter, interest me only temporarily. If, however, I occupy myself with scientific work for too long, my head becomes full and I do not feel well. On the other hand, the mere writing down of reminiscences without any pressure would not be strenuous but rather relaxing.

Of course, I do not know whether these pages will interest many people after my death, but I assume that this will be so with my son. I doubt though whether this will be the case with my grandchildren when they have reached the age to understand. That leaves my wife and my daughter Julie, as well as the family Ungethüm. Perhaps there may also be one or other of my old colleagues who may be interested in one chapter or another.

I do not want these reminiscences or any part of them to be printed. Least of all do I want them to fall into the hands of journalists. They have caused me enough anger throughout my life. Every profession has its good points and its faults. I believe that among journalists the faults predominate, at least with the majority of individuals who belong to this guild. Perhaps this will change when the "Internationale" disappears from journalism.

The following is from the Preface of the published version of the *Memoirs* by the chief Editor Professor L. Schönbauer, dated December 1950:

By chance the manuscript fell into my hands a few years ago. Since I gained the impression that its contents would arouse general interest, I approached Professor Dr. Theodor Wagner-Jauregg, the son of the great physician, with the question whether it would be possible after all to publish these pages in a suitable form. I received his agreement and it will be appreciated with what pleasure I undertook this task.

CONTENTS

Illustrations list and sources xi
Foreword by Professor Peter Berner xiii
Acknowledgements xix
Abbreviations list xxiii

Introduction 1
1. Childhood and Student Days 7
2. Early Career 23
3. Graz 1889–93 43
4. Return to Vienna 55
5. The Professorial Board 73
6. Wagner-Jauregg's Forensic Activities 83
7. The War and its Aftermath: Freud and Wagner-Jauregg . . 101
8. Wagner-Jauregg's Contribution to the Study of Cretinism 117
9. The Campaign for Goitre Prevention Through Iodised Salts 137
10. Wagner-Jauregg and Fever Therapy 151
11. Later Years 179
12. Wagner-Jauregg – The Final Chapter 195

Appendix 207
Index 211

The illustrations appear between chapters 7 and 8

Illustrations List and Sources

1. Pencil drawing of Wagner-Jauregg. (In Wagner-Jauregg's archives at the Institut für Geschichte der Medizin der Universität Wien.)

2. Introductory Note left by Wagner-Jauregg with his *Memoirs*, asking that they should not be published, with a translation and the Editor's introduction to the published *Memoirs* explaining why the request was not heeded overleaf.

3. Wagner-Jauregg as a young man. (From the Bildarchiv des Instituts für Geschichte der Medizin der Universität Wien.)

4. Wagner-Jauregg and his son Theodor (b. 1903). (From the Bildarchiv der Oesterreichischen Nationalbibliothek, Wien.)

5. Wagner-Jauregg portrait photograph. (From the Bild-Archiv der Oesterreichischen Nationalbibliothek, Wien.)

6. Bust of Wagner-Jauregg in the forecourt of the University of Vienna. (Photograph by R.T. Housden.)

7. Lecture Hall of the Second Psychiatric Clinic at the General Hospital Vienna (formerly the Chapel of the Vienna Asylum.)

8. The Vienna Asylum (Irrenheil-Anstalt in Wien) (1858). Woodcut after a drawing by C.A. Reinhardt. (From the Bildarchiv des Instituts für Geschichte der Medizin der Universität Wien.)

9. and 10. Schottengymnasium, Vienna. The school at which Wagner-Jauregg spent the last two years of his schooldays. (Photographs by R.T. Housden.)

11. Plaque on the house in the Landesgerichtsstrasse in the ninth district of Vienna where Wagner-Jauregg spent most of his adult life. (Photograph by R.T. Housden.)

12. Wagner-Jauregg with disciples and staff at the Second Psychiatric Clinic at the General Hospital, 1927. (From the Bildarchiv des Instituts für Geschichte der Medizin der Universität Wien.)

13. Malaria blood sampling under Wagner-Jauregg. (From the Bildarchiv des Instituts für Geschichte der Medizin der Universität Wien.)

14. Lecture Hall at the Institute for General and Experimental Pathology where lectures were accompanied by projected illustrations. (From the Bildarchiv des Instituts für Geschichte der Medizin der Universität Wien.)

15. Salomon Stricker (1834 – 98), Director of the Institute for General and Experimental Pathology. Teacher and later patron of Wagner-Jauregg. (From the Bildarchiv des Instituts für Geschichte der Medizin der Universität Wien.)

16. Richard von Krafft-Ebing (1840 – 1902), Professor of Psychiatry and Director of Psychiatric Clinics at Graz and Vienna, whom Wagner-Jauregg succeeded in both posts. (From the Bildarchiv des Instituts für Geschichte der Medizin der Universität Wien.)

17. Maximilian Leidesdorf (1818 – 89), successor to Meynert at the First Psychiatric Clinic and teacher of Wagner-Jauregg. (From the Bildarchiv des Instituts für Geschichte der Medizin der Universität Wien.)

18. Theodor Meynert (1831 – 92), neuroanatomist, Professor of Psychiatry at the University of Vienna and Director of the First and later the Second Psychiatric Clinic. (From the Bildarchiv des Instituts für Geschichte der Medizin der Universität Wien.)

19. 500 Schilling banknote with Wagner-Jauregg's portrait issued in 1953. (This photograph first appeared in a note by R. Underwood in *Psychiatric Bulletin*, 1992, 16: p. 777.)

20. 50 Schilling banknote with Freud's portrait issued in 1986. (This photograph first appeared in a note by R. Underwood in *Psychiatric Bulletin*, 1992, 16: p. 777.)

21. 2.40 Schilling stamp with Wagner-Jauregg's photo, issued in 1957.

22. 3 Schilling stamp with Freud's photo, issued in 1981.

23. Wagner-Jauregg portrait photograph. (From the Bild-Archiv der Oesterreichischen Nationalbibliothek, Wien.)

24. Karl Stürgk, *Graf* (1859 – 1916), Prime Minister of Austria from 1891 to 1916. (From the Bild-Archiv der Oesterreichischen Nationalbibliothek, Wien.)

25. Alexander Girardi (1850 – 1918), Austrian Comedian. (From the Bild-Archiv der Oesterreichischen Nationalbibliothek, Wien.)

Foreword
by Professor Peter Berner

There are several reasons which justify the writing of biographies of personalities who are or were believed to have made an essential contribution to the welfare or progress of mankind. In this respect it is first of all necessary to determine the objective value of the achievements under discussion. However, it is equally important to examine the part played by the subject in their realisation: were the ideas that led to his successes completely new and original or did he seize upon and pursue notions and concepts current at the time which later proved to be successful? Moreover, biographical studies can also provide insight into the characteristics marking those personalities who are responsible for extraordinary achievements. Finally, the value of such investigations may lie in their didactic consequences: from them we may learn how ideas prove successful, how lack of success and disappointments are borne without discouragement, and how to retain the flexibility to pursue new paths on the strength of unexpected results.

It seems a good idea for biographers who are not directly active in the field of the subject of the biography to investigate the state of things. Those belonging to the same professional group are in danger of seeing the personalities and work of those described in the light of their own ideas and perceptions, and thus of laying stress on matters in a way that could prejudice an objective evaluation. For this reason, it is welcome that the present biography was not written by a professional colleague of Wagner-Jauregg. On the other hand, it might be useful to add to it an accompanying commentary by a psychiatrist who himself witnessed the successes of malaria therapy, and who can supplement his own opinion by personal recollections received from some of Wagner-Jauregg's former patients and from a number of his disciples, particularly Hoff and Stransky. This Foreword should be seen in this light.

Considering the questions mentioned above to which biographical research should give an answer, it is first necessary to discuss the objective value of Wagner-Jauregg's achievements. These were in three fields: the study of cretinism and goitre prophylaxis; the reform of legislation regarding the insane; and the development of malaria therapy. There can be no doubt about Wagner-Jauregg's achievements in the first two fields. The measures resulting from them are still successfully and widely practised. They have become, as Magda Whitrow rightly remarks, so commonplace that one often forgets that they were initiated by Wagner-Jauregg. The significance of malaria therapy, the use of which has become superfluous as a result of the introduction of penicillin, is a different matter. Because of this the question has recently been raised by experts in psycho-pharmacotherapy whether the development of malaria therapy was really worthy of the award of the Nobel Prize. In this connection stress is laid, perhaps justifiably, on the fact that during the last decades certain pharmacotherapies for psychiatric diseases have produced results quite comparable with the successes achieved by malaria therapy for paralytics, yet those who initiated them were not honoured with the award of the Nobel Prize. The opinion that certain achievements have not been sufficiently recognised does not however justify lowering our respect for those who received a fitting honour. The proven value of malaria therapy, which at the time helped a large number of paralytics and encouraged the development of other somatic therapies for psychiatric disorders, is not diminished by the critical objections mentioned, nor by the fact that Wagner-Jauregg's therapy was later replaced by penicillin.

That Wagner-Jauregg made fundamental contributions to the progress of psychiatry can hardly be denied. Proofs of this are persuasively set out in Magda Whitrow's biography. However, what is the position regarding the role of his achievements in the history of ideas? To answer this question one has to remember that around the middle of the nineteenth century, Austrian university psychiatry had broken away from the ideas of the romantic movement in favour of the assumption of a somatic cause of psychiatric disorders. The pursuance of this concept soon led to the division into a *pathological–anatomic* and a *descriptive* movement. The former, whose most eminent representative was Meynert, tried to relate psychiatric diseases to certain localised cerebral lesions; the latter, which had among its members Leidesdorf and Krafft-Ebing, aimed at studying these disorders on the basis of clinical observations. The 'descriptors' accused the pathological–anatomic school of pursuing a 'brain mythology' by precipitate development of hypotheses and, moreover, of neglecting the care of their patients. Wagner-Jauregg received his psychiatric training in the descriptive school which, no doubt, was decisive in making him base his scientific investigations always on well-described observations, never losing sight of the goal of an effective treatment. That he always sought this above all in the somatic field probably reflects his interest in internal medicine. His early failure to obtain a suitable post in this field prevented him from making it his professional career. His training in the field of experimental pathology was, moreover, certainly decisive in causing him to check his assumptions experimentally. The story of Wagner-Jauregg's life shows that personal observations stimulated him in his researches and that he did not simply seize on ideas which he came across in the literature. For this reason, his great achievements in the field of biological psychiatry may be considered as original in the true sense of the word. That Wagner-Jauregg, following on his observations, searched the literature for similar experiences, and that the history of medicine showed that other physicians had made similar observations without having pursued them subsequently, does not alter the matter.

The strategy to proceed from observation to the formation of hypotheses, to check these experimentally, and then to convert them into therapeutic practice, led to Wagner-Jauregg's successes in the field of goitre and cretinism research as well as in malaria therapy. His reform of insanity legislation was based on a similar procedure: personal experience led to the recognition of weak points in the regulations for admission and detention, as a result of which mistakes and abuses occurred. To avoid these and protect psychiatrists from false accusations, he laid the groundwork for a corresponding improvement of the legal position. In contrast to these achievements, Wagner-Jauregg's reflections on genetics and eugenics derive essentially from pursuing the theories of degeneration maintained by Morel and Lombroso. They produced nothing basically new and represent a questionable facet of his scientific work, since they can be related to his German/nationalistic point of view. Without doubt these are at the root of his antisemitic stance, which – although it never led to ignoble actions – can be documented in the story of his life. Occasionally attempts have been made to blame Wagner-Jauregg's scepticism regarding psychoanalysis on his antisemitism. This is not justified for two reasons: first, Wagner-Jauregg's treatment of his Jewish colleagues shows that he was never led by racist prejudices in judging their achievements; second, his personal relation with Freud, which is treated in more detail in Magda Whitrow's biography, conflicts with such a hypothesis. Wagner-Jauregg's sceptical view of psychoanalysis may more easily be explained by his roots in the *descriptive* school which was critical of the precipitate formation of generalising theories by the *pathological–anatomic* school. Freud was brought up in the spirit of the latter by Meynert; it was not surprising, therefore, that Wagner-Jauregg considered Freud's psychoanalytical theory a great speculation. This may be illustrated by an anecdote told by Hoff. Shortly after Wagner-Jauregg received the Nobel Prize he travelled with Hoff and Schilder to a meeting. Suddenly Wagner-Jauregg said to his Senior Assistant who was a psychoanalyst: 'You look sad, Professor Schilder. But don't worry. You too will one day receive the Nobel Prize – but for literature!'

Research into the psychology and psychiatry of genius has again and again shown that, in most cases, only those who were abnormal in some psychological or spiritual sense produce outstanding work. Was Wagner-Jauregg one of those or one of the few who, despite their normality, produce outstanding feats? Portrayals of his personality suggest the latter; they describe him as outgoing, quiet, humorous and conscious of his responsibility. His patients emphasised his understanding and his confidence-inspiring bearing, as well as the modesty of the fees he charged; his colleagues especially stressed his tolerance of their interests, even if occasionally he could not forbear to make a sarcastic comment, as in the anecdote told earlier. In his professional career, he showed exemplary impartiality and tact in fulfilling many responsibilities, particularly as Dean of the Medical Faculty and as a Member of the Senior Health Council – evidence of a well-integrated personality. Ernst Kretschmer, in his book on men of genius, characterises them as those whose work is governed by an overriding idea. In this respect, Wagner-Jauregg just falls short: although there is no doubt about his devotion to work, he never exaggerated the value of ideas. Otherwise he would not always have put them aside during those periods when his competence brought upon him other tasks. Nevertheless, the story of his life suggests that much in him was not as balanced as it appeared from the outside. The strange relationship with the two women who played a part in his life, or the fact that for years he did not tell his son that he was his father are pointers in that direction. Wagner-Jauregg never commented in detail on these problems neither in personal communications nor in the written papers he left. This reserve which extends to all his personal life raises the question whether inner conflicts played a part in his successes. Perhaps he devoted himself to his scientific interests and the performance of his professional duties so tenaciously because they enabled him to conquer the problems of his personal life. If this is correct, then he also would be an example of those hypotheses which postulate that extraordinary feats are achieved by the union of talent and psychological problems.

The fundamental key to the life of Wagner-Jauregg is his insistence that reason must take precedence over sentiment – that, expressed in Stransky's terminology, the '*noopsyche*' must keep the '*thymopsyche*' in control. Even if it must remain uncertain as to how far his emotions were determined by inner conflicts or caused by his unquestionably lively nature, he always proved that he was well able to control them. This capacity helped him to meet critics and opponents with factual, rather than emotional, arguments and to produce his retorts with a strength of temperament which gave them the necessary force without shooting over the target. He treated the negative results of his investigations in a similar way: instead of dropping them with disappointment, he tried to look for the reasons for his failure in order to resume his research with new assumptions. The way in which Wagner-Jauregg subordinated his feelings to reason should no doubt be an example for all scientists to follow. With respect to the question of how far mankind in general is capable of being led by reason and higher values, he was, however, much too optimistic. For example, when he thought that national socialism would abandon its persecution of the Jews, he certainly greatly overestimated the extent of what his collaborator Economo described as 'progressive cerebration'. That he did not conceal his disappointment when he realised this, speaks for the integrity of his personality which was never questionned by those of his students who were persecuted by the National Socialists.

Wagner-Jauregg's life illustrates how intelligence, combined with acute observation and great reserves of energy and self control, enabled him to avoid speculative mistakes, and to achieve extraordinary successes. It is to Magda Whitrow's credit to have described these interrelated aspects of his work for the first time in a comprehensive, factually objective biography which is also exciting to read.

ACKNOWLEDGEMENTS

I owe a great debt of gratitude to Professor W.F. Bynum, who not only introduced me to the history of medicine and particularly the history of psychiatry, but supported me in my study of the work and life of Wagner-Jauregg in every possible way. Indeed this biography would never have been written without his advice and encouragement. It was Professor Helmut Wycklicky, formerly Director of the Institut für Geschichte der Medizin der Universität Wien, who put me in touch with many of those who knew Wagner-Jauregg and who guided me to discover much about the life of the great physician. I am most grateful to him. It was he who introduced me to the co-editor of Wagner-Jauregg's *Memoirs* (*Lebenserinnerungen*, Wien: 1950) Frau Dozent Dr Marlene Jantsch, who generously gave me much time and was good enough to show me many photographs and to talk to me about the subject of the *Memoirs* which she helped to edit. Through Professor Wycklicky I heard of Professor Theodor Wagner-Jauregg, Wagner-Jauregg's son, and of his step-grandsons Dr August and Ing. Ernst Ungethüm, the sons of Wagner-Jauregg's stepdaughter Mela, with whom I was in constant correspondence from 1987 and whom I had the good fortune to meet personally. I am very sad that all three died recently before this biography was completed. My gratitude to them is immeasurable. My husband and I travelled to Switzerland especially to meet Professor Theodor Wagner-Jauregg where he lived in retirement in Zofingen and spent a delightful day with him. I met the two Ungethüm brothers on visits to Vienna in 1987 and 1989, and both received me most courteously. Unfortunately, I can never repay my debt to them, particularly to Dr August Ungethüm, who allowed me to look through a large trunk of documents in his possession, which he had inherited from his step-grandfather. He generously allowed me to take these to the Institut für die Geschichte der Medizin der Universität Wien where they can now be consulted. Unfortunately, also Dr S.L. Last, who heard Wagner-Jauregg lecture and was much impressed by his personality, is no longer alive to receive my thanks. Although much incapacitated by a stroke he kindly granted me an interview and talked about Wagner-Jauregg.

My gratitude is due to Dr Godelieve van Heteren who succeeded in getting me a copy of Wagner-Jauregg's *Memoirs* of which no copy could be found in this country. Wagner-Jauregg probably wrote them in his old age and in a note, which Professor Theodor Wagner-Jauregg kindly presented to me, he said that he did not want them to be published. Above all he did not want them to get into the hands of journalists. He hoped, however, that some of his colleagues and members of his family might find them interesting. Professor L. Schönbauer, the historian of medicine, felt that they ought to be published, and Wagner-Jauregg's son, Professor Theodor Wagner-Jauregg, gave permission for this. Professor Schönbauer invited Frau Dozent Dr M. Jantsch to assist him in the task of editing. Inevitably my biography, particularly the early chapters, is based on Wagner-Jauregg's reminiscences. I am indebted to Professor Paul Roazen, the author of the biography of Helene Deutsch, for much helpful advice in connection with the chapter on Freud and Wagner-Jauregg; also to Dr Henry Rollin for his help, particularly with the same chapter and for his kindness in agreeing to write an appendix to this biography. I have also received helpful advice on problems that have arisen during my research on the life and work of Wagner-Jauregg from Dr Michael Hagner, Philip Housden, Dr Michael Waugh and Professor Mark Micale; my special thanks are due to Dr Renate Hauser-Birkett.

I should like to thank the staff of the Wellcome Institute for the History of Medicine and the Wellcome Library, especially Sally Bragg, and the staff of the Institut für die Geschichte der Medizin der Universität Wien, particularly Frau Inge Schidla, and also Dr Judith Bauer and Dr Karl Sablik, for their help and support. My thanks are due to the Librarians and staff of the Royal Society of Medicine, the Royal College of Surgeons and the Austrian Institute, London, for allowing me to make use of their resources, and to Dr Kurt Mühlberger of the Universitätsarchiv der Universität Wien for enabling me to see the archives relating to Wagner-Jauregg. The following Austrian archives have also generously responded to my many queries and I am greatly indebted to them: Wiener Stadt- und Landesbibliothek (Senatsrat Mag. Herwig Würtz); Wiener Stadt- und Landesarchiv (Oberarchivrat Doz. Dr Peter Csendes and Archivrat Dr Helmut Kretschmer); Oesterreichisches Staats- und Stadtarchiv (Hofrat Dr Lorenz Mikoletz); Karl-Franzens Universität Graz (Mag.Dr Alois Kernbauer); Sigmund Freud Gesellschaft (Frau Mag.Inge Scholz-Strasser); Schottengymnasium der Benediktiner in Wien (Dr S. Paulus Bergener). I should also like to thank the Secretary of the Nobel Committee for letting me see the documents relating to the award and Mrs Gunnel Ingham for translating them into English.

I am most grateful to Professor Peter Berner, who recently retired from the directorship of Wagner-Jauregg's Clinic, for so kindly writing the Foreword, and to Sir Paul Girolami, Chairman of Glaxo Holdings plc, for arranging financial support toward publication from his Company.

Last, but not least, I want to thank my husband Professor Gerald J. Whitrow for his patient support and invaluable help during the seven years of my research and the writing of this biography, without which my work could not have been completed.

The author gratefully acknowledges permission from the Editors of *History of Psychiatry*, *Medical History* and *Psychiatric Bulletin* to use material by her originally published in those periodicals.

Magda Whitrow

Abbreviations used in Bibliographies

Akad. Wiss. Wien. Akademie der Wissenschaften in Wien.
Allg. Z. Psychiat. Allgemeine Zeitschrift für Psychiatrie.
Am. J. Med. Sci. American Journal of the Medical Sciences.
Am. J. Neurol. Psychiat. American Journal of Neurology and Psychiatry.
Am. J. Psychiat. Neurol. American Journal of Psychiatry and Neurology.
Ann. Chim. Phys. Annales de chimie et de physique.
Ann. Med. Psychol. Annales medico-psychologiques.
Arch. Derm. Syph. Archives dermato-syphiligraphiques.
Arch. Exp. Path. Pharmakol. Archiv für experimentelle Pathologie und Pharmakologie.
Arch. Int. Med. Archives of Internal Medicine.
Arch. Klin. Chir. Archiv für klinische Chirurgie.
Arch. Neurol. Archives de neurologie.
Arch. Psychiat. Archiv für Psychiatrie.
Berl. Klin. Wschr. Berliner klinische Wochenschrift.
Brit. Med. J. British Medical Journal.
Bull. Acad. Nat. Med. Bulletin de l'Academie Nationale de Medicine.
Bull. Hist. Med. Bulletin of the History of Medicine.
Compt. Rend. Acad. Sci. Paris. Comptes-rendus de l'Academie des sciences de Paris.
Dermatol. Wschr. Dermatologische Wochenschrift.
Deut. Nervenheilk. Deutsche Nervenheilkunde.
Deut. Z. Chir. Deutsche Zeitschrift für Chirurgie.
Edinburgh Med. J. Edinburgh Medical Journal.

J. Am. Med. Assoc.   Journal of the American Medical Association

J. Labor. Clin. Med.   Journal of Laboratory and Clinical Medicine.

J. Nerv. Ment. Dis.   Journal of Nervous and Mental Diseases.

Jahrb. Psychiat. Neurol.   Jahrbücher für Psychiatrie und Neurologie.

Klin. Wschr.   Klinische Wochenschrift.

Med. Jahrb. Wien.   Medizinische Jahrbücher, Wien.

Med. Klinik.   Medizinische Klinik.

Mitt. Lebensmitt.   Mitteilungen für Lebensmittelforschung.

Monatsschr. Gesundheitspflege.   Monatsschrift für Gesundheitspflege.

Monatsschr. Psychiat. Neurol.   Monatsschrift für Psychiatrie und Neurologie.

Münch. Med. Wschr.   Münchener Medizinische Wochenschrift.

Neurol. Zentralbl.   Neurologisches Zentralblatt.

Oesterr. Zentralbl. Juridische Praxis.   Oesterreichisches Zentralblatt für juridische Praxis.

Psychiat. Bull.   Psychiatric Bulletin.

Psychiat. Neurol. Wschr.   Psychiatrisch-neurologische Wochenschrift.

Rev. Med. Suisse.   Revue medicale de la Suisse.

Rev. Med. Suisse Romande.   Revue medicale de la Suisse romande.

Schweiz. Med. Wschr.   Schweizerische medizinische Wochenschrift.

Sitzungsber. Akad. Wiss. Math. Naturwiss. Cl.   Sitzungsberichte der Akademie der Wissenschaften, Mathematisch-naturwissenschaftliche Classe.

Therap. Monatshefte.   Therapeutische Monatshefte.

Wien. Klin. Wschr.   Wiener klinische Wochenschrift.

Wien. Med. Blätter.   Wiener medizinische Blätter.

Wien. Med. Presse.   Wiener medizinische Presse.

Wien. Med. Wschr.   Wiener medizinische Wochenschrift.

Wien. Z. Nervenheilk.   Wiener Zeitschrift für Nervenheilkunde.

Z. Physiol. Chem.   Zeitschrift für physiologische Chemie.

Zentralbl. gesamte Neurol. Psychiat.   Zentralblatt für die gesamte Neurologie und Psychiatrie.

Zentralbl. Med. Wiss.   Zentralblatt für die medicinischen Wissenschaften.

Zentralbl. Nervenheilk.   Zentralblatt für Nervenheilkunde.

INTRODUCTION

In an article on 'Wagner-Jauregg and psychotherapy' in 1958, E. Stransky, a devoted assistant, relates that a few years previously a colleague from an English-speaking country confessed to him that he knew a lot about Freud, but had just heard the name of Wagner-Jauregg for the first time. It is true that in the English-speaking world today his name is known to very few medical men. How is it that Julius Wagner-Jauregg, the Austrian physician who was awarded the Nobel Prize in 1927, is all but forgotten now, even in his own country, unlike his contemporary and fellow student, Freud, who has become a household name all over the world? In his lifetime he received many honours, besides the Nobel Prize, and was one of the best-known psychiatrists, but his great achievements have either been superseded or become so much part of medical practice that they are no longer thought of in connection with his name. Malaria therapy for the treatment of general paralysis of the insane, for which he was awarded the Nobel Prize, is no longer used because this late stage of syphilis is hardly ever seen now as antibiotics can prevent that dreaded disease. The role of the thyroid in cretinism and its prevention by the use of iodine which he did so much to advocate have become well established. Wagner-Jauregg's work for the care and protection of the insane has been largely forgotten, because his ideas and recommendations have become part of the Austrian legislation and are now taken for granted.

Although there exists no biography of Wagner-Jauregg (1857–1940), from the many accounts of the man and his work written by pupils and assistants, there is no doubt that he must have been a very remarkable man. Sir Karl Popper CH, FRS, the eminent philosopher of science, who had occasion to visit him, was much

1

impressed by his personality and thought him very human. A British psychiatrist, Dr S.L. Last (1902–91), who attended Wagner-Jauregg's lectures in Vienna, calls him 'a very striking man – of huge stature with strong features and a powerful personality'. He once described his appearance to an artist friend who, on hearing the description, was able to draw a recognisable sketch. E. Stransky (1877–1962), who later became one of his assistants and attended his lectures when a student, emphasised the strength his appearance exuded even as a young professor. His thick black hair was short-cut; he had a thick black moustache that curled at the ends and thick black eyebrows over deep-seated eyes. He looked more like a forester than an academic, and used to dress like one on excursions into the countryside. According to his son, Wagner-Jauregg's appearance was reminiscent of a peasant in his Sunday outfit. His city clothes were very conservative, usually consisting of a white, wide-collared shirt with a wide black bow-tie and a dark-blue suit. His tailor had a piece of cloth ready to make a suit exactly like the previous one when Wagner-Jauregg gave the order over the telephone. His black hat was wide-brimmed and in winter the collar of his coat was turned up. He was so completely conservative that his dress did not change throughout his adult life, making him a recognisable figure in Viennese society. It is said that the policeman directing the traffic at the junction Wagner-Jauregg had to cross on the way from his apartment to the Clinic, saluted and stopped the traffic when he approached so that he could get across without waiting.

Although Wagner-Jauregg did not like international meetings and seldom attended them – he called them 'church fairs' – he was a regular attender at meetings of the Vienna Medical Society and of the Senior Health Council. Reports of these meetings leave no doubt as to the strength of his personality. He had the ability to make decisive contributions. Ellenberger quotes Burghard Breitner (b. 1884) who relates how Wagner-Jauregg at a meeting of the Vienna Medical Society 'crushed him against the wall like a fly'. Sometimes if the discussion became too lively, he stood up and was 'like the rock against the overpowering force'. If the issue was getting too involved, he would intervene and get some order into the proceedings. He seemed to be able 'to pour oil on troubled waters', with the result that the majority of those present would come to an agreement and go home satisfied.

In an address to a meeting commemorating Wagner-Jauregg's

death, O. Albrecht spoke of him as a giant in body and spirit. When he entered a room, he said, all those present felt as if in the shadow of a titan. Paul de Kruif, who wrote a chapter on Wagner-Jauregg in his book *Men Against Death*, likened him to a 'piece of granite rock'. I.P. Karplus (1866–1936), one of his assistants, described him as 'straight as a candle and as if chiselled in stone'. All the portraits and photographs of him that survive recall a very strong personality.

Despite his granite-like appearance and his gruff, sometimes rude, manner, he was a kind and generous man. Helene Deutsch (1884–1982), who was an assistant at his Clinic during the First World War, described him as a warm, fatherly man and very kind-hearted. He became a great figure in her life. Another of his assistants also emphasised his kindness to his pupils and to his collaborators. Yet another spoke of his 'golden humour' and of his 'double portion' of sound human understanding. He was no seeker after popularity and would not bow to authority. He had a deep moral feeling of responsibility and a touching modesty which was as much a part of his nature as was the dignity of his appearance.

One only need look through the list of his publications to realise his unusual capacity for work. In his *Memoirs* he tells how during his student days, in contrast to his fellow students who during university vacations went on holiday and had a good time, he continued to study and prepare himself for his examinations. According to his son, he possessed enormous power and strength, both physical and mental. He had great wisdom, a sure sense of what was essential, sound judgment, humour and wit and an indestructible calmness. He inspired great confidence, not only in his patients, to which his deep voice contributed.

Stransky tells of his caustic wit which was always very much to the point – he could be very sarcastic at times. Many of his sayings became proverbial and many anecdotes have been told, of which Theodor, Wagner-Jauregg's son (1903–92), mentions two. On one occasion, during Wagner-Jauregg's ward round there was considerable commotion at one corner of the ward. A patient was screaming 'Something has got to be done!' Wagner-Jauregg asked 'What has got to be done?' whereupon the patient shouted 'Either you lick my arse or I will shit into the bed.' Wagner-Jauregg replied: 'Then the latter will have to happen.' The other anecdote relates to an incident involving a simple Viennese who was brought into the Clinic because of mental confusion. Wagner-Jauregg asked him 'Do you know where you are?' The patient replied: 'I am in the

Psychiatric Clinic.' Wagner-Jauregg: 'Do you know who I am?' The patient: 'You are the professor.' Wagner-Jauregg: 'Very good', and, pointing to the assistants standing around him, 'Can you tell me who the gentlemen in the white coats are?' 'All Jews' was the reply (which was true). Wagner-Jauregg: 'You see; gentlemen, the patient is fully clear about his environment. There is no question of disorientation.'

In answer to an enquiry by a Viennese daily, popular with women, on the dangerous age of man, Wagner-Jauregg replied 'The dangerous age of man lasts from his birth to his death.' Another anecdote, related in an article of reminiscences of Wagner-Jauregg, tells of a visitor to the Clinic who asked Wagner-Jauregg 'Excuse me, Sir, where are the madmen?' Wagner-Jauregg pointing outside replied 'The madmen are out there', and then turning to the door of the ward, he said 'in there are the sick men'.

Although Wagner-Jauregg had a sharp tongue, he was not overbearing. He could take umbrage if anyone tried to make fun of his scientific endeavours, and he was ambivalent as far as opposition was concerned. He did not really like it, although he would not admit this. On the other hand, he valued those of his students who were able to produce independent work. He once said of a former assistant with his usual sarcasm 'He was only my student'. In his *Memoirs*, Wagner-Jauregg mentioned his disdain for those who only imitated their masters.

He was natural and friendly towards even the most junior doctors, but he liked to keep his distance and no one was allowed to forget this. He was very tolerant of his scientific colleagues, always encouraging them and promoting their interests; many of them have written in praise of his sterling qualities. Stransky recalled two incidents which showed Wagner-Jauregg's magnanimity: on one occasion, he allowed Stransky to submit a paper for his lecturer's status although he disagreed with his thesis; on another he did not take amiss the fact that Stransky disagreed with his evidence when called as an expert witness in a criminal trial.

He was unconventional, not only in his appearance, but also in his mental attitude. If he was reading some voluminous work which he needed to consult, he would tear it up into parts and only keep the part in which he was interested, in order to read it while travelling.

One of his assistants commented on Wagner-Jauregg's fearlessness and absolute devotion to truth. He looked at his own work critically and was always ready to abandon his own method in favour of someone else's which he considered superior. In forensic matters his main interest was not the psychiatric aspect of a criminal action, but the understanding of the criminal person. His outstanding characteristics were goodness and humanity, so that his students learnt even more by his human example than through his science.

Although Wagner-Jauregg had great energy and a firm will, he had considerable understanding of the human weakness of his patients, and from the beginning of his career he aimed at the relief of man's suffering. He had a very strong social conscience which was reflected in his choice of those whom he made the object of his therapeutic endeavours: paralytics who were thought to be incurable, cretins who represented extreme forms of lack of intelligence, and criminals who stood outside society. In later years, his interest in heredity and eugenics demonstrated his concern for the future of society. Although, as a scientist, he was attracted by clinically important problems, it was not knowledge for its own sake that he sought but knowledge that might benefit humanity. Throughout all his scientific work his constant endeavour was to find a successful therapy.

BIBLIOGRAPHY

This introductory chapter is largely based on memoirs, reminiscences, biographical essays and obituary notices. They are listed below in alphabetical order.

Albrecht, O. Memorial meeting. *Wien.Med.Wschr.*, 1940, 90: no. 44, 844.

Benedek, L. *Wien.Klin.Wschr.*, 1937, 50: 491–494.

Breitner, Burghard. *Hand an zwei Pflügen*. Innsbruck: Inn Verlag, n.d., pp. 222–224.

de Kruif, Paul. *Men against Death*. London: Jonathan Cape, 1933.

Ellenberger, Henri F. The discovery of the unconscious. London: Allen Lane, 1970.

Hitzenberger, Anneliese. *Die Frau*, 9.3.1957, p. 10.

Hochstetter, F. *Akad.Wiss.Wien*, Almanach for 1941, 91:197–203.

Hoff, Hans. *Oesterreichische Nobelpreisträger*. Wien: Wilhelm Frick, 1961, pp. 83–94.

Karplus, I.P. *Wien.Med.Wschr.*, 1932, 82: no. 12, 373–375.

Kauders, O. *Wien.Klin.Wschr.*, 1947, 59: 130–132.

Last, S.L. *Psychiatric Bulletin*, 1989, 13: p. 402.

Lesky, Erna. *Dictionary of Scientific Biography*. New York: Charles Scribner's Sons, 1976. Volume XIV, pp. 114–116.

Pötzl, O. *Wien.Klin.Wschr.*, 1940, 52: no. 40, 1–4.

Roazen, Paul. *Helene Deutsch. A psychoanalyst's life*. New American Library, 1985, pp. 127, 183.

Schmeidel, Hermann von. *Tagespost* (Graz), 11.3.1937.

Stransky, E. *Selbstbiographie*. M.S. held at the Institut für Geschichte der Medizin der Universität Wien; *Wien.Klin.Wschr.*, 1957, 69: 177–8; *2nd International Congress for Psychiatry*, September 1957, Vol. 1, 47–50.

Thury, Elizabeth. *Weltpresse*, No. 100, 1951.

Wagner-Jauregg, Julius. *Lebenserinnerungen*. Ed. L. Schönbauer and M. Jantsch. Wien: Springer Verlag, 1950.

Wagner-Jauregg, Theodor. *Mein Lebensweg als bioorganischer Chemiker*. Stuttgart: Wissenschaftliche Verlagsgesellschaft m.b.H., 1985.

ONE

CHILDHOOD AND STUDENT DAYS

Little is known about Julius Wagner-Jauregg's childhood. He was born on 7 March 1857 in Wels, a small town in Upper Austria, the son of Adolf Johann Wagner (1816–94) and his wife Ludovika, née Schmeidel. Half of his mother's ancestors came from Lower Austria, the other half from Silesia, while his father's family was of Silesian origin. On his mother's side one branch originated from a family Ranzoni in Treffinne near Cannobio, the Italian part of Lago Maggiore. Giuseppe Carlo Antonio Ranzoni was born there in 1711 and is reputed to have fled northwards over the Alps after killing his brother in the course of a fight caused by jealousy. He married in Tulln, Lower Austria, the widow of a chimney sweep and carried on this occupation until his death in 1773. Wagner-Jauregg's son believes that the slightly dark and foreign aspect of his father's face and his lively temperament may be traced back to this Italian forebear.[1]

Julius's paternal grandfather, who was born in 1785 and died in 1873, was a cloth-maker, but following the invention of the mechanical weaving loom his son had to choose another career. After studying jurisprudence and politics (the family must have been reasonably well-off), he entered the Civil Service. He first worked at Wels, where his son Julius was born, and later in Stein, near Krems, a small town on the Danube.

Julius was the second of four children, having one brother and two sisters. The death of his mother from tuberculosis in 1867, soon after the birth of the youngest child, destroyed a happy family life. The daughters were sent to a convent, but the boys stayed at home. Julius went to school at Krems until 1872 when his father was

7

moved to the Department of Finance in Vienna.* For his last two years at school he went to the famous Schottengymnasium, a high school for boys, which had been founded in 1807 as part of a Benedictine Abbey. As a result of the overhaul of the educational system by Count Leo Thun (1811–88) during the 1850s, the school was reformed. The stress fell no longer on religion and obedience to the state, but on training students to engage in research at the university, and the atmosphere was full of respect for learning. The Benedictines who taught there did not foster clericalism, and included in the curriculum natural science as well as several years of Latin and Greek. The Schottengymnasium, which was one of the three best schools in Vienna, was popular among the nobility as it was less secular than the other two boys' grammar schools. Among the 36 pupils in Wagner-Jauregg's class who passed the final examination there were six titled boys. Thirteen of the class, including Wagner-Jauregg, were awarded distinctions. Julius's final certificate shows that the marks obtained by him in religion, Greek, German, history and geography, physics, natural science, mathematics and propaedeutics were excellent; his mark in Latin was praiseworthy; and in behaviour he was described as exemplary.[2] At the Krems grammar school he also studied French and Italian and read much in these languages. He taught himself English at a later date. There are no letters or reminiscences of Julius's school days nor of his early childhood, so that we do not know how much he was affected by his mother's death. In his *Memoirs* he gives a fairly detailed account of his career only from the time he enrolled at the university in 1874.[3]

During his school and student days Julius lived with his family in an apartment in an inner suburb of Vienna. His father had remarried, probably about the time of the move to Vienna. It has not been possible to ascertain the date of the marriage of Adolf Wagner to his second wife, Karoline Schurz (1834–1915), but Julius must have been on good terms with his stepmother because many years later she became a godmother to his daughter.

In his old age Wagner-Jauregg could not remember how he came to study medicine although there was not a single medical man in his family. His father wondered whether he would take up the

---

* Shortly before his retirement as a senior civil servant, Adolf Wagner was ennobled and he chose the title von Jauregg. When in 1918 titles were abolished in Austria his son was granted permission to retain the additional name by adding it to his family name.

subject because whenever his son came across a dead animal he cut it open to see what was in it. Adolf would have liked his son to take up philosophy with a view to becoming a high school teacher, possibly because that course of study would have taken only three years instead of the five needed for medicine – and would thus have been far less costly. However, as his son received a grant from the penultimate year at high school to the end of his university career, that consideration ceased to be of importance. In any case, Julius's father did not exert any pressure on him and right up to his matriculation Wagner-Jauregg remained uncertain whether to take up philosophy or medicine. What decided the issue in the end was the news that two of his schoolmates who had done less well than he did opted for medicine. He followed suit and enrolled in the medical faculty at the University of Vienna in October 1874 at the age of 17½.

The Vienna Medical School was founded by Gerard van Swieten (1700–72), a disciple of Hermann Boerhaave (1668–1745), who was summoned to Vienna by the Empress Maria Theresa (1717–80). He reorganised medical studies and established clinical teaching on a sound basis of observation. The School flourished and in 1784 Joseph II (1741–90) founded the General Hospital (the buildings of which still exist), the Maternity Hospital, the Asylum and the Foundlings Home. The revolution of 1848 led to a new order in medical studies. Freedom to teach and learn was granted and medical courses were reformed, largely due to the efforts of Ludwig Freiherr von Türkheim (1777–1846), the founder of the Vienna Medical Society. Only one medical degree – that of doctor of medicine – was to be recognised. The new constitution of the Medical Faculty led to the exclusion of General Practitioners (who because of their number – 437 in Vienna in 1848 – had been in complete control of the Medical Corporation), and to Faculty Members taking charge of the administration of the Medical Faculty. Even before 1848 great developments had taken place in the Vienna Medical School, with new departments and institutes being created. The founding of an Institute of Pathological Anatomy under Carl von Rokitansky (1804–78) led to another revival of medical science in Vienna. Through the joint endeavours of Rokitansky and Josef Skoda (1805–81) the Vienna Second Medical School became, in Virchow's words, 'the Mecca of Medicine'. Rokitansky is reported to have performed more than 85 000 autopsies, developing pathological anatomy into the first reliable tool of diagnosis. He was supported in his work by Skoda who coded Rokitansky's results of post-mortem examinations thereby laying the foundations of modern diagnostics. Not only Rokitansky and Skoda, but also the anatomist Josef Hyrtl (1810–94) and the dermatologist Ferdinand von Hebra (1816–80) attracted pupils in great numbers. A German physician, Adolf Kussmaul (1822–1902) who had come to Vienna to attend a medical course in 1849, has described some of his experiences.[4] He witnessed about 300 clinical autopsies performed by Rokitansky who recorded his findings by dictation. According to Kussmaul, Rokitansky looked very kind and reliable. He found Hebra's courses on skin diseases the most instructive of the many to which he subscribed, being both very clear and often entertaining. In the summer they began at 7 a.m. and lasted until 9 a.m.

When Wagner-Jauregg began his studies, Rokitansky had retired and so had Hyrtl who was forced to retire prematurely because of an eye disease which eventually led to blindness. Wagner-Jauregg much regretted having missed Hyrtl's lectures which were said to have been very entertaining. Numerically his year was a weak one: there were only about 145 undergraduates. Half of them were Hungarians, who at the time were still able to study in Vienna, although some years later the Hungarian government decreed that medical men with an Austrian degree were not allowed to practise in Hungary. Wagner-Jauregg made friends with three fellow students somewhat older than himself, perhaps because intellectually he was much more mature and a more serious student than most of his contemporaries.

One of those was Adolf Lorenz (1854–1946) who became an eminent orthopaedic surgeon and remained a life-long friend. During the first year Wagner-Jauregg attended not only lectures on physics, chemistry, zoology and mineralogy, but also on anatomy, and he took part in dissecting exercises. The lectures on physics given by an eminent physicist, Victor von Land (1838–1921), who made no attempt to hide his boredom in having to teach medical students and pharmacists, were not popular. Students preferred the anatomy rooms and Wagner-Jauregg enjoyed the chemistry lectures which he attended regularly.

Regulations regarding the times when examinations could be taken had been changed just before Wagner-Jauregg commenced his studies. Until then, all examinations had to be taken at the end of the five years needed for the study of medicine with the result that many medical students attended lectures rarely or not at all. They did not bother to do a great deal of studying during the first four years, only applying themselves during the fifth year when they attended some of the lectures which they had missed in the earlier years. It had often taken students 10 years to get their degree, but under the new regulations the three preliminary examinations in zoology, botany and mineralogy could be taken during the first two years and the first principal set of examinations, the first 'Rigorosum'* at the beginning of the fifth semester, i.e. in the first part of the third year.

Wagner-Jauregg had not at first realised that the regulations had been changed, but as soon as he did he entered for the examination in botany. As the date for this was postponed for some reason, he thought he would enter for the mineralogy examination at the same time, although he only had one week to prepare himself for the latter. He passed both with distinction during the second semester, having had a good grounding in these subjects at school. He then concentrated on zoology. The lectures were delivered by Ludwig K. Schmarda (1819–1908), an 'agreeable old gentleman' who preferred to speak on edible animals. He had lost his Chair in Prague in 1848 because he was involved in the political unrest of the time ('just as today', commented Wagner-Jauregg, writing in the thirties). He was eventually appointed an ordinary professor in Vienna in 1862, where his lectures were stimulating, if a little out of date. Wagner-Jauregg took his preliminary examination in zoology in the autumn of 1875 at the beginning of his second year and passed with distinction. He was now free to concentrate on the first Rigorosum. As in England and other European countries, this included the basic medical sciences, consisting of three examinations: a practical examination in anatomy, another in physiology, and theoretical examinations in anatomy, physiology, chemistry and physics.

During the winter semester of his second year Wagner-Jauregg spent most of his working time in the dissecting room. Already during the winter semester of his first year (no dissecting was done during the summer semester) he had done some dissecting on bones and extremities, whereas in the second year he had to dissect complete corpses. Conditions, as far as dissecting material was concerned, were ideal. The number of medical students was small and there were plenty of cadavers available, so that each student was assigned four corpses during that semester. Groups of four students

---

*Similar to the first MB.

were assigned to one corpse. However, since there were lazy medical students who preferred to find their amusements elsewhere, Wagner-Jauregg had the opportunity of working on at least six whole cadavers during that winter semester and they were recently deceased bodies, not those that had been lying in carbolic acid for months.

The second most important subject during the second year was physiology, for which the lectures were given by Ernst von Brücke (1819–92), an outstanding scholar, student of the famous physiologist Johannes Müller (1801–58). To Wagner-Jauregg's regret the lectures were not enlivened by experiments, whereas he was greatly stimulated by the practical exercises in histology. During these he learnt to handle a microscope and to prepare specimens so as to be able to study the microscopic structure of organs. Although Brücke came to the Laboratory from time to time, practical tuition was in the hands of four senior medical students.

Wagner-Jauregg entered for the first Rigorosum at the earliest possible date and achieved a record by passing the theoretical examination in his fifth semester. He obtained distinctions in all subjects having had an advantage over his colleagues in that he remained in Vienna during the long vacations, whereas the other Viennese went on holiday and the remaining students went home so that they had little chance of furthering their studies. He worked mornings and afternoons and often did his reading in one of the Vienna parks, hoping to cure the haemoptysis from which he was suffering as a result of a tubercular lung infection, as his family was not able to afford to send him to a health resort. One wonders whether he had inherited some weakness from his mother, who died of tuberculosis at an early age. To get some exercise in the evenings he often ran from his home in the Lederergasse in an inner suburb of Vienna up to the Kahlenberg or Leopoldsberg (two hills in the surrounding countryside) or to some other place in the Vienna woods, distances of about four miles covered in an incredibly short time. He was a great walker and a good all-round sportsman. Except to the east, Vienna is surrounded by beautiful hilly country which is easily accessible. The eighth district, where Wagner-Jauregg lived, is particularly close to the Vienna woods, so for a young man this excursion would have presented no problem. Nowadays a new road leads up to the hills which has made them much more accessible, but alas, has robbed them of much of their attraction.

Having passed the first Rigorosum, Wagner-Jauregg was now ready to turn to clinical studies. He attended lectures on internal medicine by Heinrich von Bamberger (1822–88) during four semesters, on surgery by Theodor von Billroth (1829–94) during three semesters and by Johann von Dumreicher (1815–80) during the fourth.

Heinrich von Bamberger, who came from the Prague Medical School, was called to Würzburg after working three years in Vienna. There he came into contact with Virchow's circle* and learnt about the foundations of cellular pathology. He was the first to include pathological chemistry in clinical study by analysing the chemical composition of body fluids, secretions and excretions, thus achieving a synthesis between clinic and laboratory. He returned to Vienna when he was appointed to the chair of internal medicine in Vienna in 1872. In each lecture Bamberger presented one or two cases and called for volunteers to examine the patient and, having been told the case history, to make a diagnosis. It was always the same few students who volunteered because most were afraid to expose their ignorance, and – needless to say – Wagner-Jauregg belonged to the group of volunteers. Afterwards Bamberger gave a most instructive formal lecture, delivered, however, in a manner that gave the impression that he was bored with the subject.

Theodor Billroth was one of the outstanding surgeons of his time. After studying at universities in Germany, France and Great Britain, he became professor of surgery at Zurich at the age of 31 and seven years later, in 1867, he was appointed to a chair in Vienna. Regarded as the founder of abdominal surgery, he was a keen follower of Lister's methods,[†] without which his great achievements, particularly in the surgery of abdominal cancer, would not have been possible. Wagner-Jauregg had been drawn to Billroth's lectures because of his reputation and his imposing personality, but he found them disappointing because they were on too high a level for medical students, being more suited to the fully qualified doctors and surgeons who always attended them. During the operations performed in the course of the lectures, the medical undergraduates saw only the backs of the assistants or the other doctors who were called 'pupils in surgery'. Once a week Billroth held a continuous lecture on some subject with the aid of many pictures, models and tables.

---

* Rudolf Virchow (1821–1902).
† Joseph Lister (1786–1869).

Johann Heinrich Freiherr Dumreicher von Oesterreicher, the other professor of surgery, who was appointed in 1849, was not on good terms with his colleague. He was very conservative and did not believe in Lister's antiseptic methods. His lectures differed markedly from those of Billroth, since his aim was to train general practitioners, not those who intended to specialise in surgery. There were no large-scale operations, only small-scale surgery. The German physician A. Kussmaul, mentioned previously, who had attended several medical courses many years before, witnessed in Dumreicher's Department the first operation carried out with chloroform as an anaesthetic in place of ether. At that time the Department had no operating theatre and operations took place in the wards, often surrounded by other patients – a situation which Dumreicher found greatly upsetting. Presumably these conditions had changed by the time Wagner-Jauregg attended Dumreicher's lectures as he does not mention them. From all accounts Dumreicher must have been an excellent teacher.

During Wagner-Jauregg's period of study it was the custom for assistants to make afternoon rounds in the wards and medical students were expected to attend. Few of them actually did so, and they particularly avoided the rounds of the surgical wards. Wagner-Jauregg, however, being an exemplary student, attended these rounds and often he and another student, later Professor Gustav Gärtner (1855–1937), were the only two present. When a patient of the Clinic for Internal Medicine, who had been presented at one of the lectures, died, the professor and his students attended the *post mortem*.

During the third year of medical study several of Wagner-Jauregg's more ambitious colleagues who had influential connections were already working at various institutes on scientific research, and some even had salaried positions as demonstrators. Wagner-Jauregg was anxious to do some scientific work, but he did not think that he stood much chance as he did not know the right people. However, he happened to see on one of the boards carrying announcements that there was an opening at the Institute for General and Experimental Pathology for a third-year medical student to take part in scientific research and to assist with experiments during lectures. He immediately went to see the head of the Institute, Professor Salomon Stricker (1834–98), though with little confidence in securing the post. However, Stricker seemed to like him and was clearly impressed that Wagner-Jauregg had passed the first Rigorosum so early and so successfully and he appointed him. In retrospect Wagner-Jauregg considered this to have been of the utmost importance for his future career.

Stricker was an outstanding scholar. Wagner-Jauregg had already attended some of his lectures in his fourth semester – they were normally attended in the fifth and sixth semesters – because his attention had been drawn to them by colleagues. He found them lively and stimulating as Stricker was a lecturer who strove to establish contact with his listeners instead of adopting the 'Jupiter-like manner of Bamberger or Billroth who always remained at a distance from their audience'.[5] At the time Stricker's lectures were the only ones in which animal experiments were carried out. Indeed, few experiments were being done in the other institutes and certainly not during lectures.

Stricker's Institute was a creation of Rokitansky who had realised that the methods of anatomy alone could not solve pathological problems. When Wagner-Jauregg joined the Institute it had only existed for a few years. Stricker advised him regarding the scientific publications he ought to read and gave him the corpses of experimental animals for dissection so that he would learn about animal anatomy. He had to assist in the preparation of experiments to be performed during lectures and in the experimental work at the Institute. Stricker also gave him a subject on which to work under his direction: 'The accelerating nerves of the heart'. This work involved several animal experiments which for more than a year occupied the young Wagner-Jauregg, who was acquiring some skill in vivisection. In the course of these investigations it was found that they contradicted the findings of a researcher at the laboratory of Karl Ludwig (1816–95) at Leipzig, but Wagner-Jauregg was able to prove that his own results were correct. The paper describing this work was published in March 1878 under both Stricker's and Wagner-Jauregg's names.[6] In July 1879, a second paper describing experimental work by Wagner-Jauregg was published under the title 'Contributions to the knowledge of the respiratory activities of the nervus vagus'.[7]

Already during his period at the Institute, a new phase was looming in Wagner-Jauregg's career. At that time, medical students were obliged to work for a year at a military hospital as volunteers, though they were allowed to continue with their studies during their free time. This period of military duty was usually taken during the fourth year of the medical course. Although it could not be taken earlier, it could be postponed until a later stage in the course, or even after graduation. Wagner-Jauregg was anxious to join the navy as a volunteer medical cadet, but to be able to do this he had to be accepted for military service. Moreover, not having reached his twenty-first year at the time, he had to have his father's permission, and his father was reluctant to give this because he feared that the Russo-Turkish war would involve Austria. If his son waited until he was obliged to join up, the clouds on the political horizon might possibly have disappeared. However, he eventually agreed and Wagner-Jauregg entered the service on 1 October 1877, his naval ambitions bringing him four advantages which reconciled his father to this step. First, medical naval cadets worked at the military hospital in the ninth district, close to his parents' home and to the University and the Institute; whereas some of the other cadets were located at a hospital in the third district which made it difficult for them to continue their studies. Second, the expenses of naval cadets were paid by the State which, in view of his father's position as a high civil servant, would not have happened otherwise in his case. Moreover, he received a lump sum towards the necessary equipment. Third, he received a monthly salary during the time of service of which he was very glad because his father allowed him only a small amount of pocket money. Fourth, as a naval cadet he was able to wear a waistcoat and naval jacket which he much preferred to the army jacket which was closed right up to the chin.

No one troubled much about the military training of medical men. They were called twice into a courtyard of the military hospital, made to stand in formation and march a little; they were also taught how to salute and how to deliver military messages. That was the extent of their military training!

Wagner-Jauregg was first assigned to the department of a staff-surgeon major whose goodwill he enjoyed because his parents knew him through a friend, Baron Kremer (1828–89). Due to his influence, Wagner-Jauregg's time in the service was made a great deal easier. General conscription had not long been introduced in Austria and the authorities were at a loss to know what to do with the medical students, of whom about 120 were standing around the two military hospitals. One of the cadets was entrusted with the task of writing the monthly report of the First Military Hospital. For this purpose, he had to collect certain statistical data, such as the movement of patients, etc.; otherwise he was free of duties. Wagner-Jauregg was assigned to be his assistant, but since the compiler was afraid that someone might discover that he had very little to do, he did not introduce Wagner-Jauregg into the secrets of the monthly report. Instead he sent him every month to the meteorological station on the 'Hohe Warte', a hill in the environs of Vienna, to copy the temperatures, barometer readings and other meteorological data concerning the past month, which had to be attached to the report. All Wagner-Jauregg had to do during the whole month was to spend one morning at the meteorological station, and he was thus free to attend university lectures and continue his work at Stricker's Laboratory. With his military partner he remained friends to the end of his life.

Sadly, this idyllic life as assistant to the compiler of the monthly report only lasted for a few months. At the Congress of Berlin Austria had received a mandate to take over the administration of Bosnia and Herzegovina and to keep an occupational army at Novibazaar. At the end of July 1878 Bosnia and Herzegovina were eventually occupied, but the task was not as easy as had been expected. The Muslims in these two provinces put up a heavy resistance, resulting in a guerilla war in difficult mountainous country and costing Austria considerable expenditure and great losses in men until the revolt was quelled after about three months. All the doctors serving at the military hospital were sent to the front and their duties had to be taken over mainly by the military cadets and a few assistant doctors who were doing their one-year voluntary service. Wagner-Jauregg was at first assigned to the surgical department which was run by an unpleasant and odd man whose methods of treatment had cost many a healthy young soldier his life. Later the prosector of this hospital became the head of the department, but he cared very little for how it was run. About 100 of the injured were entrusted to the care of the cadets although they knew nothing of surgery. All they were able to do was to substitute the dirty bandages with clean ones; this they did every day until the injured were transferred to another hospital and a new intake of wounded troops arrived. They could have learned a great deal had there been anybody to tell them or to show them what to do. On one occasion the head of the department felt the ambition to perform an operation. With some commotion an injured man was brought in: a projectile had got impacted in a wound and needed to be extracted. After the surgeon had poked around the wound for some time without finding the projectile his ambition was satisfied and he gave up. After that incident no further operation was performed.

The military commandant of the hospital one day decided to

show his appreciation of the work done by the cadets. Leading them into the cellar where there was a great barrel of wine, he opened the tap which was to remain open until he gave the sign for it to be closed. He had asked each cadet to bring some drinking vessel, and Wagner-Jauregg and two colleagues had managed to get hold of one holding a litre which they filled three times and emptied. By the time the commandant called a stop, after about 15 to 20 minutes, Wagner-Jauregg had imbibed a litre of strong wine in a very short time and the others had drunk no less. When they left the cellar they felt rather hot and did 'something very sensible'.[8] They took the horse-tram to the public bathing beach and cooled down through a longish stay in the waters of the Danube.

According to regulations, at the end of their service the cadets had to take an examination on military subjects on which lectures had been given during the year, but which few of them had attended. A pass in this examination entitled the candidate, once he had taken his doctor's degree, to be promoted to assistant physician in the Reserve. Although some of the cadets had done some work, most had postponed their studies until the end of their period of service and because of their heavy duties during the last three months they had had no time to devote to them. The students revolted and decided not to enter for the examination. Wagner-Jauregg was chosen as their spokesman and he conveyed the cadets' decision to the medical commandant of the hospital who was greatly annoyed. A compromise was arrived at: if the students agreed to sit for the examination, they would be assessed with great leniency. Indeed they all passed, although most of them were quite ignorant!

In September 1878 the period of service ended and Wagner-Jauregg was able to return to civil life. Despite his military duties he had been able to attend lectures at the eye clinic and the obstetric clinic during the winter semester, and attend Bamberger's clinic for internal medicine and Billroth's surgical clinic during the summer semester. He missed most lectures on forensic medicine because of the time spent in Stricker's Laboratory. He greatly benefited from the lectures on surgery by F.F. Salzer (1827–90), which he was able to attend in both semesters as they were held in the evening.

At the obstetric clinic, in addition to attendance at lectures, students had to do practical training, for which they had to be at the clinic in the evening since 'most deliveries take place at night',[9] according to Wagner-Jauregg. They were divided into groups of six which were allowed to practise in turn, and there was a room with some beds where students could sleep in their clothes when nothing was happening. They were called when a delivery was to take place, and were allowed to examine women in childbirth who were in the delivery room. In each of the three obstetric clinics about 3000 deliveries took place per year so that there were plenty of patients to practise on. 'Having children was still the custom then'[10] remarks Wagner-Jauregg in his *Memoirs*.

In his last year at the University Wagner-Jauregg attended obligatory lectures on internal medicine and surgery. He remained faithful to Bamberger as he was not attracted by the lectures of the other professor in internal medicine, A. Duchek (1824–82), who was only interested in auscultation and percussion. He attended lectures at the eye clinic of Ferdinand von Arlt (1812–87) which he found very instructive.

The time had arrived for him to prepare himself for the second and third Rigorosum. He had passed the first main examination in record time, but with the second and third things were more difficult. Because of his work in Stricker's Laboratory he was not able to concentrate on his studies as much as he would have liked. He got on reasonably well with his preparation for the second Rigorosum, which consisted of practical examinations in pathological anatomy and internal medicine, and a theoretical examination in pathological anatomy, general pathology, pharmacology and internal medicine. Having passed the two practical examinations, he put his name down for the theoretical examinations on a Monday, and was called for the Tuesday of the following week. On the previous Saturday he went down with a mild attack of measles, but he nevertheless intended to present himself for the examination. However, when the professors heard of his illness they would not allow him to do so. Wagner-Jauregg suspected that his parents had somehow managed to let them know. However, he took the theoretical examination a week later, on 29 January 1880, and passed all three examinations with distinction. When it came to the third main set of examinations, it was necessary to attend courses for the practical examinations, given by the assistants of the Professors. He also heard more lectures on obstetrics by J. Späth (1823–96), a congenial, sensitive Tyrolean, who in 1848, as a member of an academic guard company, had taken part in the defence of South Tirol against the Italians.

Wagner-Jauregg recalled an interesting episode during one of Späth's lectures which for the first time acquainted him with the

Semmelweiss affair. Talking about puerperal fever, Späth came to speak of the work of Ignaz Philipp Semmelweis (1818–65). He became quite emotional when, with tears in his eyes, he defended himself against the accusation that he had taken part in persecuting Semmelweis. It is true that at first he had been against Semmelweis, but soon became persuaded that Semmelweis was right and he then took his side. The undergraduates did not understand much of the affair and had no idea of Semmelweis's fights and his important contribution to medicine. Semmelweis realised that the frightening incidence of puerperal fever at the obstetric clinic where he worked was due to the fact that students and physicians came straight from the dissecting room into the clinic and attended to patients without washing their hands. The statistics at the clinic compared most unfavourably with those at the other obstetric clinic where midwives attended to the women. Semmelweis showed that the infective material that conveyed the fever was brought by the hands of the doctors from the dead bodies. His discovery was bitterly opposed by the head of the clinic, but although it soon became accepted by other medical men in Vienna, Semmelweis's life ended tragically.

Wagner-Jauregg had already done some practical work in obstetrics, having attended a course by Späth's assistant, Friedrich Schauta (1849–1919). On one occasion, after a lecture, Späth went into the delivery room where a forceps delivery had become necessary, turned to the students and asked for volunteers. Wagner-Jauregg came forward and offered to do the operation. Späth agreed, but one of his assistants suggested that it should be performed by one of his American students. Thinking that the assistant did not trust Wagner-Jauregg, Späth reluctantly agreed. It is clear from Wagner-Jauregg's account of this incident that it greatly angered him and also his colleagues, and he was obviously glad when he passed the examination in the subject with distinction.[11]

Up to that point, Wagner-Jauregg had passed every one of the examinations with distinction and had thus become a candidate for the *Promotio sub auspiciis Imperatoris*. This was an award made to university students who passed all university examinations with distinction and had completed their school careers similarly. The award was conferred in a special ceremony at which the candidate had to make a speech and a representative of the government handed him a ring studded with diamonds and bearing the Emperor's initials. Unfortunately, in the practical examination in ophthalmology Wagner-Jauregg suffered a set-back. Although he thought he was well prepared, he only received the passmark 'satisfactory', and so his hope of gaining the Emperor's award was thwarted. He was clearly upset at the time, but as a result was not quite as disappointed when he received the same mark in the last examination, a practical examination in surgery. He blamed Billroth for his poor result. The examination consisted of two parts: first, a patient at the clinic had to be examined and the case discussed; then an operation had to be performed in the Anatomical Institute. The candidate had to draw a piece of paper from an urn on which was written the name of the operation to be performed. Wagner-Jauregg drew *Exarticulatio humeri* (disarticulation of the humerus). When it came to the examination, Billroth had forgotten the question and confused it with *Resectio humeri* (resection of the humerus). He did not allow Wagner-Jauregg to complete the operation otherwise he would have realised the error, and Wagner-Jauregg tried unsuccessfully to make him understand his error. He was given the mark 'satisfactory', but since he had already missed the chance of the special award, he did not mind. The final examination, the third theoretical one, included surgery, ophthalmology, obstetrics and forensic medicine and these he passed with distinction.

REFERENCES

[1] Theodore Wagner-Jauregg. *Mein Lebensweg als bioorganischer Chemiker*. Stuttgart: Wissenschaftliche Gesellschaft, 1985, pp. 8–23; *Die Presse*, 3.3.1957, pp. 17–18.

[2] I am indebted to Dr S. Paulus Bergener, of the Schottengymnasium der Benediktiner in Vienna, for his kindness in sending me copies of the relevant documents.

[3] Julius Wagner-Jauregg, *Lebenserinnerungen*. Ed. L. Schönbauer and M. Jantsch. Wien: Springer Verlag, 1950.

[4] A. Kussmaul. *Jugenderinnerungen eines alten Arztes*. Stuttgart: 1899.

[5] Wagner-Jauregg, op.cit. ref 3, page 11.

[6] *Sitzungsberichte der math.-naturwiss. Classe der k. Akademie der Wissenschaften*, 1878, 77: III. Abt. 103–132.

[7] Ibid. 1879, 80: III. Abt., 177–187.

[8] Wagner-Jauregg, op.cit. ref 3, page 17.

[9] Ibid. page 21.

[10] Ibid. page 19.

[11] Ibid. pages 20–21.

TWO

EARLY CAREER

W agner-Jauregg was awarded his doctor's degree on 14th July 1880 at a ceremony which was very casual and which he found most disappointing. It was held in the rooms of the Dean of the Medical Faculty, which were devoid of all decoration, in the presence of the Rector of the University, the Dean and the Registrar. He always remembered the date because the day is a national holiday in France, commemorating the storming of the Bastille.

It was now time for him to think of his future. He already had good prospects of a position in the Institute for General and Experimental Pathology where he had been working since 1876 without remuneration, although some of his fellow undergraduates who worked at other institutes received stipends for demonstrating. On 1 January 1881, Professor Salomon Stricker, the Director of the Institute, was granted permission to appoint a second assistant and Wagner-Jauregg was offered the post. Although he accepted he had no intention to remain at the Institute for long and to have an academic career in its field, since his ambition at the time was to travel and emigrate. Even in his old age he sometimes still regretted not having done so.

He had five months between the award of his degree and the start of his work at Stricker's Institute. At that time the Austrian branch of the shipping company Lloyds was engaging young doctors for one or more tours, which not only enabled them to make interesting voyages and see distant lands, but also brought them in some money to take home provided they were not spendthrifts. Moreover, he may have thought that life on board ship would be good for him and cure him of the haemoptysis from which he suffered during his student days. In his old age, Wagner-Jauregg vaguely remembered having once been on the way to the Lloyds Office in Vienna to apply for such a post, but he did not recall why nothing had come of the idea.

Another plan was much more serious, and if it had materialised it would have diverted Wagner-Jauregg's career into quite different channels. On the occasion of the wedding of the Crown Prince Rudolf to Princess Stephanie in 1881, her father, the King of the Belgians, had come to Vienna. He had persuaded the well-known explorer H.M. Stanley (1841–1904) to undertake another expedition to the unexplored hinterlands of the Congo and he wanted to engage an Austrian doctor, Emil Holub (1847–1902), who was then in Vienna working on material brought back from a journey in South Africa. Holub declined the offer. The King, however, was anxious to engage an Austrian – perhaps, Wagner-Jauregg remarks in his *Memoirs*,[1] because he would be cheaper than a member of another nationality. He therefore asked Holub to suggest a suitable candidate and Holub put a notice on the board of the medical reading room in the General Hospital. Wagner-Jauregg saw it by chance and on impulse decided to apply for the post. However, there was another candidate who had been in the tropics before, having worked for the Dutch Government in their Far Eastern colonies for two years. Wagner-Jauregg expected him to be chosen, but in the end neither candidate was given the post.

Another opportunity for emigrating presented itself towards the end of 1881 while Wagner-Jauregg was already working as an assistant in Stricker's Institute. A Protestant Missionary Society in Basle had inserted an advertisement in a Vienna medical journal for a doctor who was prepared to go to the Gold Coast, where the Society had outposts, to study the diseases which were common in those regions. In reply to Wagner-Jauregg's letter to the Society asking for details, he was told that he would have to go to England for some months to learn more about these diseases. The stay on the Gold Coast would be for six months at a salary of 2000 Marks and travelling expenses. In reply to a letter in which he agreed to the conditions but asked for some further information, he received word on 10 November 1881 that the Society had found a suitable doctor in Basle. Wagner-Jauregg wondered whether his being a Roman Catholic had prompted this decision. His suspicion was probably correct since the original letter from the Missionary Society, which was recently discovered among his papers, states that the applicant should be Protestant and sympathetic to the aims of the Mission. One wonders why he bothered to apply.

The idea of emigrating came to the fore again a year later when his application for a post at the Clinic of Internal Medicine, to which he was anxious to move, was turned down. It is strange that a man who came from Austrian peasant stock and was in many ways a typical Austrian should have been so anxious to leave his country. It is futile to speculate whether this renewed attempt to leave his native land was merely a youthful desire to see the world or due to some peculiar facet of his character. He planned to settle in Egypt where he hoped to receive considerable help through the influence of his family friend, Baron Kremer, who had made things easier for him at the Military Hospital. Baron Kremer was a diplomat and orientalist who was highly thought of in Cairo. He was the Austrian member of an international Finance Commission which supervised Egyptian finances since the Viceroys had mismanaged the economy and run up heavy debts abroad. However, once again Wagner-Jauregg was unlucky. Even before he had asked for Baron Kremer's assistance the political scene in Egypt had changed. During 1882 Arabi-Pasha, the fanatical Egyptian nationalist, had become Minister of War and had eventually assumed dictatorial powers. The British bombarded Alexandria on 11 July, defeated Arabi-Pasha at Tell-al-Kebir on 13 September and occupied Egypt. This put an end to the international Finance Commission and thus to the activities of Baron Kremer. Reflecting on this episode in his old age, Wagner-Jauregg realised that he had not really pursued his plans for emigrating to Egypt very seriously. There were several branches of medicine in which he had not gained enough experience, for example dermatology, paediatrics and ear, nose and throat diseases. Moreover, he had not troubled to learn English and had otherwise postponed decisions, so that he wondered later whether subconsciously he had realised that nothing would come of the project.

His attempts at finding work in distant places having failed, Wagner-Jauregg remained in Vienna and continued to work in Stricker's Institute, though he would have preferred to work in internal medicine. However, he became very skilled in performing animal experiments and was often called upon to assist other researchers. There arrived at the Institute Dr Josef Lakarski (1854–1924), an assistant to the Professor of Pharmacology, August Vogl (1833–1909), who was anxious to be selected for the chair in pharmacology at Cracow. Up to that time Lakarski had only written two papers on pharmacognosy (Wagner-Jauregg called them 'dried herb essays'[2]), but Cracow demanded evidence of some experimental work. Stricker was reluctant to take him into the Laboratory, but Wagner-Jauregg was on good terms with Lakarski and persuaded Stricker to let him work there. He claimed that Lakarski would be no trouble because he would look after him, they were to work together on prussic acid, the plan having been worked out by Wagner-Jauregg who was to conduct the animal experiments. All Lakarski had to do was to pay for the laboratory animals and to distil the prussic acid, yet the work was published in 1881 under Lakarski's name alone.[3] The result was no epoch-making discovery, but it nevertheless revealed something of interest. Prussic acid, injected into an animal, kills it within seconds. The circulation is arrested, blood pressure drops immediately to zero and life ceases. The experiments revealed, however, that if prussic acid is given in extremely minute doses, the opposite effect is achieved, namely a considerable increase in blood pressure. On the strength of this paper Lakarski was appointed a professor in Cracow. He never showed any gratitude to Wagner-Jauregg; indeed, when some time later Wagner-Jauregg applied for the post of assistant at Bamberger's Clinic, Lakarski supported the other candidate.

Another project also caused some annoyance. A Pole from the Russian part of Poland, Theodor von Openchowski (1854–1914), wished to do some experimental work in Stricker's Institute to help him obtain a professorship in Russia. Stricker suggested that he should investigate 'The measurement of blood pressure in the pulmonary circulation' under the supervision of Wagner-Jauregg. All the difficult animal experiments were planned and carried out by Wagner-Jauregg since Openchowski was not able to carry out the intricate surgical part of these. The research was completed successfully and as Openchowski had only assisted, Wagner-Jauregg expected that at least his name would appear as co-author of the resulting paper since Openchowski,[4] apart from paying for the animals, had only assisted in the work. This suggestion enraged Openchowski, who insisted that only his name should appear as the author because he needed to show that he was capable of distinguished work. Stricker supported him as he was glad to have researchers from abroad at his Institute since they not only paid the costs but enhanced its reputation. The matter was settled by Wagner-Jauregg's contribution being redeemed by the payment of

150 Gulden. However, there were hard words exchanged between them. Openchowski got his professorship, but as Wagner-Jauregg remarks in his *Memoirs*[5] 'Famous he did not become and he has been dead a long time.'

In later years Wagner-Jauregg looked back critically to the animal experiments carried out at the time. In retrospect they seemed to him very cruel indeed and he wondered at the peculiar intellectual attitudes of researchers who valued the benefits that might accrue to humanity so highly that they were prepared to justify the ghastly tortures inflicted on dogs, cats, rabbits and other animals. The experiments were made with the aid of curare, an extract from the bark of South American trees, which paralysed all voluntary muscles, including those responsible for respiration, but not the heart. During an experiment, like the one to investigate the blood pressure in the pulmonary circulation, artificial respiration was effected by introducing a canula and fixing it into the trachea, injecting curare, and rhythmically inflating the lungs of the experimental animal with the aid of bellows. The whole thorax and the front ribs were then opened by dissecting the sternum, while a canula was introduced into the carotid artery and another into a branch of the pulmonary artery – the most difficult part of the operation. These were connected to a kymograph which registered the pressure in the systemic and pulmonary circulation. Wagner-Jauregg thought that it redounded to the credit of the animal protection societies to have protested against research involving such cruel experiments. In several countries the use of curare for this purpose became prohibited by law.

Wagner-Jauregg carried out various operations, such as irritating or cutting single nerves or the spinal cord, injecting various poisons, to study their effect on the systemic and pulmonary circulation. One of these experiments impressed Stricker so much that he used it regularly in his lectures; it involved a study of the blood pressure. This is considerably lower in the pulmonary circulation than in the systemic. If, however, artificial respiration is stopped so as to cause asphyxiation, then the pressure not only increases in the systemic circulation but also in the pulmonary, so much so that it reaches the pressure in the former and eventually exceeds it as the latter begins to fall due to asphyxiation. The left ventricle of the heart is increasingly inflated because it can no longer expel blood against the great resistance created by the contraction of all blood vessels in the systemic circulation, thus causing the blood to dam up in the lungs and the right ventricle to do more work to empty itself.

Nevertheless, it is not enlarged to the same extent as the left ventricle because through the contraction of the small blood vessels and capillaries little blood reaches it through the systemic veins. For medical students the performance of such experiments on mammals was very instructive.

Another piece of research concerning blood pressure involved a claim by the Swiss physiologist Adolf Fick (1829–1901) that the systolic pressure in the left ventricle was less than the pressure in the aorta. To Wagner-Jauregg this seemed paradoxical, since the blood from the left ventricle flows into the aorta and not the other way round. Fick explained his assertion by arguing that through the contraction of the ventricle the blood acquires an increased velocity and can thus overcome the aortic pressure on the valves. Stricker was very enthusiastic about the subject and repeated Fick's experiment in his lecture. However, there were voices of criticism and Wagner-Jauregg was asked to report on the matter at the regular evening seminars which were held at the Institute. He found to Stricker's surprise that Fick's discovery was a delusion, caused by the measuring instruments which he had used. Stricker took the matter very seriously and considered Wagner-Jauregg's attitude as a kind of rebellion against the authority of the Institute. He asked Wagner-Jauregg to provide experimental proof of his claim, which he succeeded in doing. Although Stricker was a passionate fighter, he valued truth above anything and he was prepared for Wagner-Jauregg to publish his result. However, Wagner-Jauregg, anxious to retain Stricker's good will, refused. In general, he was not anxious to publish unless the work seemed to him to be important. He had not asked for his name to appear on the paper of Lakarski's work, as he considered his help an act of friendship.

It is not easy to speculate on Wagner-Jauregg's relationship with Stricker. He clearly had great admiration for his chief but he did not always see eye to eye with him and, although Stricker supported him throughout his career, he may not have had a great liking for the younger man. Stricker must have been an excellent lecturer. To improve his delivery he had taken lessons with a well-known actor. He not only described experiments but, as we have seen, performed them in his lectures. He endeavoured to develop microscopic projection to make it usable for medical teaching and also to improve electrical projectors. Not only did Stricker teach general and experimental pathology, but he also tried to train his assistants and students in the art of teaching. In the evening seminars at his Institute, those taking part had to report in turn on progress in their different fields of research. After each lecture Stricker not only discussed the methodology and technique of research, but also the art of lecturing, including even the right way to stand and to move. Wagner-Jauregg attributed his own lecturing technique to what Stricker had taught him in these seminars.

On the other hand, Wagner-Jauregg had great misgivings about the future of the Institute which had been created by Carl von Rokitansky, the great pathological anatomist. According to Wagner-Jauregg, he had made the mistake of choosing for posts in pathology physiologists who were not familiar with the problems of the subject (Stricker had received his training from Ernst von Brücke, who had been a student of the great physiologist Johannes Müller). Unfortunately, at the time there was no one in Austria with a knowledge of both general pathology and experimental method. In Wagner-Jauregg's opinion a specialist in general pathology ought to have developed an interest in bacteriology which was already flourishing at the time and was soon to cause a revolution in the whole field.

He soon discovered that Stricker was not the man to do this. He was once asked by Stricker to report at one of the evening seminars on a number of researches into the causes of tuberculosis. (This was just before Koch's discovery of the tubercle bacillus.) These researches dealt with various experiments to induce an illness similar to tuberculosis. Wagner-Jauregg took the view that tuberculosis was probably due to a live organism, but Stricker violently opposed this view and was supported by others, particularly his other assistant Arnold Spina (1850–1918), whom Wagner-Jauregg called Stricker's evil spirit. In his opinion, Spina had a bad influence on his chief because he was not concerned with the truth but with obtaining results that would please his senior. Stricker was opposed to the idea of the tubercle bacillus because its discoverer, Robert Koch (1843–1910), enjoyed the support of Julius Cohnheim (1839–84) in Breslau with whom Stricker had been having a bitter, almost personal, scientific dispute regarding the role of tissue cells in inflammation. Because of his refusal to admit the existence of the tubercle bacillus, Stricker would have nothing to do with bacteriology. However, as a result of the intervention of Dr Emil Amrusch (d. 1919), a friend of Wagner-Jauregg, a 'covered withdrawal' from the fight against the tubercle bacillus by Stricker's Institute was set in motion.

Fearing that the chair for experimental pathology might be

discontinued, Wagner-Jauregg, with Stricker's agreement, turned to internal medicine and spent his free time at the Clinic for Internal Medicine, directed by Bamberger, where he hoped to obtain a post as an assistant. The first assistant, Joseph Vincenz Kauders (1850–1916), planned to relinquish his position in the near future and he favoured Wagner-Jauregg's application. Bamberger's attention had been drawn to Wagner-Jauregg and he asked him to confirm a statement made in a French journal refuting the assertion by some French researchers that fuchsin reduces the separation of albumen from the urine in kidney disease, and may even cause it to disappear. To carry out this work, Wagner-Jauregg had to make a daily quantitative analysis of the albumen and urea in the urine of two kidney patients in the Bamberger Clinic from October 1880 to February 1881. Although this investigation proved nothing, Bamberger requested Wagner-Jauregg to write an article on the fuchsin tests for the *Wiener Medizinische Blätter*. Wagner-Jauregg did not wish to do this as the tests had been quite inconclusive, but Bamberger had promised that article to the Editor of the periodical and insisted that the tests be written up. Wagner-Jauregg had to comply, but refused to let it appear under his name. This led to the unusual situation that the first article in the issue of that journal for 7 April, 1881, entitled 'On the effect of fuchsin on the albumen-urea in Bright's disease'* was published as a 'Communication from the Medical Clinic of Professor v. Bamberger in Vienna' without the name of an author. Wagner-Jauregg admitted that this was not a clever move on his part and did not improve his prospects of becoming an assistant at the Clinic. Pride, not vanity, he said, had always been a fault of his, but at the same time his greatest virtue.[6]

There is an interesting sketch of Bamberger in Wagner-Jauregg's *Memoirs*.[7] In these he describes him as an excellent diagnostician who had written some outstanding larger works, including a textbook on cardiac diseases and one on abdominal diseases. He was highly educated, well versed in philosophy, and his lectures were polished and informative. Nevertheless, his listeners were made to feel that the subject bored him: his eyes were half-closed, he never looked at the audience and did not seek contact with his listeners, as Stricker always tried to do. He did not care about the scientific work done by his assistants: instead of encouraging them, he usually

---

* Richard Bright (1789–1858).

discouraged them. Wagner-Jauregg found an interesting case in the Clinic, a patient in whom the pulse of the pulmonary artery could be felt. With the aid of Knoll's polygraph he obtained curves which showed this pulse very clearly; moreover, they were most unusual. He continued to observe these symptoms which he also found in two or three other patients. During his round of the Clinic, Wagner-Jauregg drew Bamberger's attention to this patient and showed him the curves, expecting him to show some interest. Bamberger listened, but then without a word continued on his round. The patient died later and during the post-mortem it was found that the upper lobe of the lung had become caseous as the result of tuberculosis and no longer covered the pulmonary artery. Having been discouraged by Bamberger, Wagner-Jauregg did not publish anything on this case.

It is probably not surprising that Wagner-Jauregg did not get the post at the Bamberger Clinic, but unexpectedly the chance occurred of an appointment as assistant at the Second Clinic for Internal Medicine. In the spring of 1882, the head of that Clinic, Adalbert Duchek, died and a violent struggle ensued regarding his successor. One party wanted to appoint Ernst von Leyden (1832–1910) of Berlin who had a great reputation; Bamberger supported a student from his time at Würzburg, Karl Gerhardt (1833–1902), who was professor there. After lengthy negotiations the choice fell on Hermann Nothnagel (1841–1905), professor at Jena, whose work until then had been theoretical and experimental rather than clinical. Bamberger's son, who was a friend of Wagner-Jauregg, suggested that he should apply for the post of assistant at the clinic which was then becoming vacant. Wagner-Jauregg did so and expected to be appointed, since Nothnagel owed his appointment to Bamberger, but to his disappointment Nothnagel informed him that he had already appointed Rudolf von Jaksch (1855–1947) with whose father he had worked in Berlin. That was the end of Wagner-Jauregg's prospect of a post in a clinic for internal medicine, and he had already told Stricker that he did not wish to continue his appointment at the Institute after the end of 1882. Thus he thought of emigrating to Egypt, as recounted earlier, but fate decreed otherwise.

Since his appointment as assistant at Stricker's Institute, Wagner-Jauregg had been reasonably well-off. He had to be careful, but since he still lived with his parents, he was able to join colleagues for meals at a nearby restaurant or in the early evenings in a coffee house where they played cards. One day two of his colleagues suggested that he ought to apply for the post of assistant at the

Psychiatric Clinic of the Landesirrenanstalt (the Asylum of Lower Austria) under Professor Max Leidesdorf (1818–89) which was becoming vacant as one of the assistants was leaving. There he would not only receive the same salary as at the Institute, but also free accommodation and full board. He would also have plenty of spare time to prepare for his plans to emigrate. On the following day he went to see Professor Leidesdorf with the two papers he had produced at the Institute. He was appointed and his fate was sealed, although strangely enough he had never thought of becoming a psychiatrist. He had never been to a lecture on psychiatry and had hardly ever looked at a textbook on the subject as psychiatry was not a compulsory subject in the medical syllabus at the time. However, as he reflected in his *Memoirs*[8], this hasty decision had done neither him nor psychiatry any harm.

Wagner-Jauregg was due to start work at the First Psychiatric Clinic on 1 January 1883. Since he knew nothing about psychiatry, he began already in October to attend the rounds at the Clinic which Leidesdorf held daily at 8.30 a.m. and to immerse himself in the textbook on psychiatry by Heinrich Schüle (1840–1916). He had once before held the book in his hand when his father's brother had been taken ill with progressive paralysis in 1877 or 1878 while Wagner-Jauregg was doing his military service, and he was called upon to help when his uncle had a paralytic fit. On that occasion he made the acquaintance of the distinguished professor of psychiatry Theodore Meynert (1833–92), who was called in as a consultant to his uncle.

Wagner-Jauregg actually began work at the Clinic on 23 December 1882. His circumstances changed radically: he not only had his own room but he was also allowed to use another room which lay between his and that of his colleague, the first assistant. From his window he had a lovely view of the large park around the main building of the asylum and beyond that over a great part of the city as far as the 'Prater', a large open space with a famous amusement park. Until then he had shared a room at his parents' home with his brother Fritz which looked out on to a small courtyard surrounded by three-storey buildings.

He ate at the Clinic where the food was plentiful and good and received a monthly salary of 57 Gulden. He found friendly company, for the medical staff – besides the two assistants, there were four assistant medical officers and two student doctors – and the administrator, a former medical man, lived in close contact. Already on the first day, which happened to be an unusually beautiful one for the time of year, they were playing bowls together out in the open in shirt sleeves after lunch until the afternoon visits.

Gradually it became clear that the post offered him favourable prospects for the future and he abandoned the idea of emigrating. He was not only assistant to the professor, but also assistant medical officer at the Clinic. The Clinic was one of three departments of the Asylum, the other two being respectively for permanently interned male and female patients. This meant that at the end of his period as assistant he could remain on the medical staff at this, or move to a similar post at another asylum in Lower Austria, and might eventually become chief physician and director. If he continued his scientific research there was also the possibility that he might become a lecturer or even a professor. He had enjoyed his work at Stricker's Laboratory and was loathe to give up research.

Soon after he began work at the First Psychiatric Clinic his position improved still further. The first assistant, Dr Raab, was appointed to a post at the Provincial Asylum at Graz and Wagner-Jauregg succeeded him. At the time the duties of the assistants were quite strenuous. There was no other medical staff at the Clinic apart from the two assistants each of whom had to be on duty every other twentyfour hours. In the morning both had to be present at the same time. At noon the assistant on duty, together with the assistant doctors of the asylum, had to go into the kitchen to supervise the food distribution; then in the afternoon until four o'clock he had to receive the patients' visitors and supply information in the lecture room, which also served as the office of the Clinic. There followed the afternoon round, and at night, the assistant on duty was often woken once or twice. There were about 150 patients in the Clinic and great care had to be taken in writing up their case histories because, when a patient was discharged or transferred to another institution, his or her case history had to be submitted to the Director who was especially anxious that it should be written properly. 'Nowadays,' Wagner-Jauregg writes in his *Memoirs*[9], 'there are many more assistants and other helpers. On the other hand, in my time it was possible to attain a Chair or become a chief physician much earlier, whereas now people are as old as the hills by the time they have achieved a position.'

During the first few months at the Clinic, Wagner-Jauregg had to familiarise himself with the subject of psychiatry, by reading textbooks and other relevant literature. The Asylum had a small library to which Wagner-Jauregg appointed himself librarian. It contained only books relating to matters connected with asylums, and he had to go to the library of the Vienna Medical Society, which at the time was housed in the building of the Academy of Sciences, for the literature that he needed to consult. His election to the Society in March 1883, on the proposal of Professor Leidesdorf, entitled him to use the library.

The facilities for scientific research at Leidesdorf's Clinic were very meagre. There was one large lecture room and a smaller adjoining room. The lecture room, in which there were six benches for the students, served also as a consulting room for those patients whose thorough examination could not be carried out in the wards; and as an office where visiting permits were issued to the patients' relatives and where they could be interviewed. The laboratory facilities consisted of a table built into a niche under a window, a microscope and a primitive microtome. There were a few cupboards where preparations could be kept and in the ante-room to the lecture room, which could be entered from the garden, there was a boarded partition for experimental animals.

Despite these meagre facilities, Wagner-Jauregg managed to do some research on brain anatomy. He examined the brain and spinal cord from bodies of paralytic patients and brains of epileptic patients who had died in the asylum and whose post-mortems he always attended. He studied whatever interested him, irrespective of whether it would lead to publication and thus further his career. He often spent a great deal of effort on problems which he dropped before completing work on them. Sometimes after he achieved a result that satisfied him he lost interest and did not get it ready for publication. It seems that he did not greatly enjoy writing. Although Leidesdorf took an interest in Wagner-Jauregg's work, he did not often advise or encourage him beyond showing him a book or an article and asking for his opinion.

His circle of colleagues at the asylum did not encourage him to engage in scientific work. They were pleasant people and evidently liked him, but they had no scientific ambition and preferred the social life. After supper they often sat in the room of one or other of the medical staff drinking beer; in the summer they sometimes amused themselves in the bowling alley. The clerical staff of the asylum, together with their wives and visitors from outside, took part in these social activities and Wagner-Jauregg found it quite hard to get away to pursue his scientific work. Sometimes he would stay with the company for an hour after supper and then go to the laboratory and work there until midnight or even later. In this way he succeeded in completing a number of researches and publishing several papers.

At the beginning of 1884 at Leidesdorf's suggestion Wagner-Jauregg carried out some experiments on animals on the effect of removing the thyroid gland, the first step in a field of research which he took up again some years later and which he pursued until the end of his active life. An account of these experiments will be given in the chapter on Wagner-Jauregg's work on cretinism. In the same year he published a paper on diseases of the spinal cord in patients suffering from paralysis, based on a clinical description and anatomical examination of a case which he had observed at the Clinic.[10] He also began to study nervous diseases, although he saw such cases at the Clinic only occasionally, and he took an interest in electrotherapy. As a result he published, together with a colleague, Eugen Conrad, a paper 'On the value of Engelskjön's electrodiagnostic examination of the field of vision',[11] in which the method of examination described by the Swede was shown to be incorrect. Another outcome of Wagner-Jauregg's electrophysiological work was a paper on a method to produce skin anaesthesia by means of cocaine.[12] Karl Koller (1851–1946) had introduced the anaesthetising effect of cocaine in eye operations. Wagner-Jauregg found that by means of electrical cataphoresis it was possible to produce anaesthesia in healthy skin by moistening the electrode used as an anode with a cocaine solution. He was anxious to show the theoretical importance, rather than the practical applicability, of this discovery because the absorption of substances through the healthy skin was still a contested question. Together with Heinrich Paschkis (1849–1923) he demonstrated that the claim by Albert Adamkiewicz (1850–1921) of Cracow that anaesthesia could be produced by applying chloroform through cataphoresis in the healthy skin was incorrect. He and Paschkis made the experiments on themselves and in Wagner-Jauregg's case they left him with a sizeable pigmented circle on his left forearm.

Wagner-Jauregg tells an amusing anecdote relating to cocaine anaesthesia by cataphoresis.[13] Edmund von Neusser (1852–1912), who later became a professor at the same time as he did, was once consulted by the King of Bulgaria because of violent neuralgic or rheumatic pain in the nape of his neck. Neusser used the cocaine method, which seemed irrational as it did not reach beyond the skin and the King had no pain in the skin. But Neusser was able to demonstrate to the King by pin pricks on the skin of the affected area that he could no longer feel any pain. The King, having – according to Wagner-Jauregg – transferred this skin insensitivity by auto-suggestion to his original pain, was cured. After that the King favoured Neusser and helped him in every way. Wagner-Jauregg comments that with some people only the irrational works, though the explanation may not have been as irrational as Wagner-Jauregg thought. If the pain was neuralgic, then introduction of cocaine into the skin might be expected to relieve it.

Already at the beginning of 1885 Leidesdorf asked Wagner-Jauregg to apply for recognition as a University Teacher (Dozent) in neurology. Wagner-Jauregg was hesitant since he had only worked in the field for two years, but Leidesdorf insisted. He heard later from Stricker that there had been a somewhat acrimonious meeting between Leidesdorf and Meynert, the head of the Second Psychiatric Clinic at the General Hospital in Vienna, regarding this application. The two had been rivals when the First Psychiatric Clinic was founded at the Asylum, a rivalry in which Meynert was victorious. In private practice, however, Leidesdorf was much more successful because Meynert was rather aggressive. However, under Stricker's influence Meynert agreed not to oppose Wagner-Jauregg's application which then went to the Board of Professors and was confirmed by the Ministry of Education on 9 May 1885.

The lectures which Wagner-Jauregg was required to give in his new position involved him in much work. In addition to these he also gave a course on neurology at the Clinic of Professor Bamberger. For this he had to get his cases with the help of friends among the assistants and more junior doctors. He recalls in his *Memoirs*[14] a case that brought him a small triumph. A patient who had suffered an injury to his head – a barrel had rolled over him as he slipped when carrying it down into a cellar – had become blind in one eye, could not speak and had no sensation on one side. Meynert and the ophthalmologist Ernst Fuchs (1851–1930) were greatly interested in the case and speculated about how these symptoms could be explained anatomically. Wagner-Jauregg had read some of Jean-Martin Charcot's (1825–93) teachings on hysteria and described the case as one of hysteria, which caused Meynert and Fuchs to smile sarcastically. However, one day this patient became very angry over a patient in the next bed and proceeded to box his ears, swearing loudly all the while. From this moment he regained his speech and his sight, and Fuchs was generous enough to tell Meynert that it seemed that in this case Wagner-Jauregg was correct.

In 1887, together with Gustav Gärtner, his successor at Stricker's Institute, he published a paper based on difficult experimental investigations on the circulation in the brain.[15] One of its most important findings was that, during an epileptic fit artificially produced by stimulating the cortex, the blood vessels in the brain are considerably enlarged. The paper was cited by many, but it did not receive the attention Wagner-Jauregg thought it deserved. It was only a preliminary communication and he felt that more details and references should have been given in a full report, which neither he nor Gärtner had the perseverance to produce. On another piece of research, an anatomical study of the spinal cord and the medulla oblongata, he only gave a brief report[16] and again did not follow it up with a detailed account of the experiments and a list of references. In the course of this work he discovered that in certain animals with a prominent tail there was an unpaired nucleus of the grey substance exactly in the centre of the medulla oblongata. He intended to publicise this in the full version of the paper which was never written. However, he passed this discovery on to a colleague without any request to refer to himself.

During the next two years he wrote four papers arising from his experience at the Psychiatric Clinic. The first[17] was a description of a case of salicylic acid poisoning accompanied by delirium which had been wrongly diagnosed as a case of Delirium alcoholicum. Examination of the patient's urine and the fact that he was constantly thirsty suggested that he was suffering from diabetes insipidus. Moreover, it was discovered that a doctor had prescribed for him Natr. salicyl. 12.0 in three doses. The effect of this was increased because of the large amount of fluid intake as a result of his diabetes. Wagner-Jauregg complained that neither the Austrian nor the German Pharmacopoeia mentioned a maximum dose of salicylic acid or its salts.

The second was a very long and detailed paper on the relationship between trauma, epilepsy and mental derangement,[18] in which a number of cases are cited where head injury had led to epilepsy and moral insanity. Another paper investigated cases of neuralgia causing insanity.[19] Wagner-Jauregg gave a detailed account of a patient suffering from a psychosis of neuralgic character, and referred to a case of Dysthymia neuralgica transitoria reported by the famous German psychiatrist W. Griesinger (1817–68). In a paper on the relationship of osteomalacia and mental derangement[20] he gave full details of five cases. He speculated on the nature of this disease which was then not only little known but the cause of which had not been discovered. (It is a form of adult rickets due to lack of vitamin D which was not discovered until 1919.) He found that there had been many more cases at his Psychiatric Clinic than at that of the General Hospital.

However, the subject that was at the back of his mind during his period at the Leidesdorf Clinic and remained thereafter his chief interest was the effect of infectious diseases on mental illness. Soon after he arrived at the Clinic he observed a case of a woman patient suffering from insanity who was cured after an attack of erysipelas. This led him to make a very thorough search of the literature to discover other incidents in which an infectious disease had had a similar beneficial effect. A detailed account of this is given in the chapter on fever therapy.

In 1887 an event occurred that was of great importance for Wagner-Jauregg's career. At the beginning of the winter semester 1887/88 Leidesdorf suffered a severe heart attack during a lecture and asked Wagner-Jauregg to continue the lecture for him. From that day until he left the Clinic in 1889, Wagner-Jauregg not only took over Leidesdorf's lectures but was also entrusted with the running of the Clinic. The Dean of the faculty, Professor Hans Kundrat (1845–93), who evidently liked Wagner-Jauregg, pointed out to him that unless he was recognised as a university teacher in psychiatry, as well as in neurology, he would not be considered for a senior academic position and he advised him to apply for recognition. This was readily granted in June 1888 since Wagner-Jauregg had already acquired considerable experience and had obtained Meynert's goodwill by supporting the Society for Psychiatry and Neurology in Vienna, of which Meynert had been a co-founder. The Society began its activities in 1868 and Meynert became its President in 1873. Already during that year differences of a personal nature between the leading members of the Society surfaced. The Director of the Asylum in Vienna, Professor L. Schlager (1828–85), resigned from the Society and Professor M. Leidesdorf relinquished the editorship of the journal sponsored by the Society. Attendance at meetings dropped, and at times only ten to twelve members were present. In 1878 Leidesdorf together with his two assistants left the Society for personal reasons. H. Obersteiner (1847–1922), who wrote a history of the Society from its foundation in 1868 to 1918,[21] is somewhat silent on the causes of the disagreements, but as will appear in a later chapter these leading representatives of the psychiatric profession did not get on with one another. (Wagner-Jauregg seems to have been an exception.) However, Leidesdorf rejoined the Society in 1882 and no doubt he encouraged Wagner-Jauregg to support it.

During his last year as an assistant at the Clinic, Wagner-Jauregg was asked by Leidesdorf to take over some work which was to cause him much time and trouble. Although Leidesdorf had retired from the Clinic, he was still a member of the Senior Health Council, an appointment that had no age limit. In that capacity he was asked to report on 'the creation of a law which would make it possible to set up asylums for alcoholics with forcible internment of dipsomaniacs.' He gave Wagner-Jauregg the whole dossier and asked him to give an expert opinion. Wagner-Jauregg wrote a 27-page report in which he advocated the setting up of two types of institution, one for curable drinkers who agreed to voluntary treatment and one for the detention of morally depraved drinkers with criminal dispositions. Furthermore he stressed that it should be made possible to certify alcohol addicts. Leidesdorf signed the report and passed it on to the Senior Health Council. A few months later he died. Eduard von Hofmann (1837–97), an expert in forensic medicine, who played a leading role on that Council, later commented to Wagner-Jauregg that he was surprised that the sick Leidesdorf had been able to write such an excellent report. Wagner-Jauregg admitted that he had written it and afterwards believed that this might have been a factor in his appointment to the Council when he returned to Vienna some years later.

After Leidesdorf's retirement Richard von Krafft-Ebing (1840–1902) was appointed his successor. Krafft-Ebing had been Professor of Psychiatry at the University of Graz and Director of the Psychiatric Clinic since 1873. A Swabian by birth, he retained his strong Swabian accent and Wagner-Jauregg found it difficult to understand him when they first met. He had studied in Zürich under Wilhelm Griesinger and at the University of Heidelberg, and worked as an assistant at the famous asylum at Illenau for four years. After spending some time as a neurologist in general practice in Baden-Baden, he decided to resume work in psychiatry and accepted a call to the University of Strasbourg, whence he moved to Graz a year later. He is best known for his textbook on sex variants *Psychopathia sexualis*.

Wagner-Jauregg doubted whether Krafft-Ebing would want an assistant who had been acting as professor and director of the Clinic for two years, and he therefore began to look for a post elsewhere. Among his papers discovered recently there is a letter from Moriz Holl (1852–1920), who was leaving the University of Innsbruck to take up a Chair in Anatomy at the University of Graz, asking whether Wagner-Jauregg would like him to intercede on his behalf regarding a vacancy at Innsbruck; there is also a letter from Stricker, dated June 1889, praising Wagner-Jauregg and recommending him for an appointment at Innsbruck. However, Wagner-Jauregg hoped very much that he might be called to the post of extraordinary professor and director of the Psychiatric Clinic at Graz which Krafft-Ebing was vacating. Although there were three other candidates, he was appointed to the vacant position in Graz towards the end of September 1889. A few days after his arrival there he had to return to Vienna for Leidesdorf's funeral. He had seen him briefly before his departure for Graz, and Leidesdorf was obviously touched and very pleased that one of his assistants should have become the director of a psychiatric clinic.

REFERENCES

[1] Julius Wagner-Jauregg. *Lebenserinnerungen.* Ed. L. Schönbauer and M. Jantsch. Wien: Springer Verlag, 1950.

[2] Op.cit. ref 1, p. 24.

[3] Josef Lakarski. Ueber die Wirkung der Blausäure auf Atmung und Kreislauf. *Med.Jahrb.Wien,* 1881, 141–160.

[4] Theodor von Openchowski. Ueber die Druckverhältnisse im kleinen Kreislaufe. *Sitzungsber.Akad.Wiss.,* *Math.-Naturwiss.Cl.,* 3 Abt., 1881, 84: 203–7.

[5] Op.cit. ref 1, pp. 25–27.

[6] Op.cit. ref 1, p. 32.

[7] Op.cit. ref 1, pp. 32–33.

[8] Op.cit. ref 1, p. 36.

[9] Op.cit. ref 1, p. 38.

[10] Julius Wagner-Jauregg. Ein Beitrag zur Kenntnis der Rückenmarkserkrankungen der Paralytiker. *Med.Jahrb.Wien.,* 1884, p. 369.

[11] Julius Wagner-Jauregg and E. Konrad. Ueber den Wert der Engelskjön'schen elektrodiagnostischen Gesichtsfelduntersuchung. *Arch.Psychiat.,* 1885, 16: no. 1.

[12] Julius Wagner-Jauregg and H. Paschkis. Ueber die durch Chloroform auf kataphoretischem Wege zu erzeugende Hautanästhesie. *Neurol.Zentralbl.,* 1886, p. 413.

13 Op.cit. ref 1, p. 41.

14 Op.cit. ref 1, pp. 46–47.

15 Julius Wagner-Jauregg and Gustav Gärtner. Ueber den Hirnkreislauf. *Wien.Med.Wschr.*, 1887, 37: no. 19–20.

16 Julius Wagner-Jauregg. Zur Anatomie des Rückenmarks und der Oblongata. *Zentralbl.Nervenheilk.*, 1886.

17 Julius Wagner-Jauregg Vermeintliches Alkohol-Delirium, diabetes insipidus, Salicylsäurevergiftung. *Wien.Klin.Wschr.*, 1888, 1: no. 38, 778–780.

18 Julius Wagner-Jauregg. Ueber Trauma, Epilepsie und Geistesstörung. *Jahrb.Psychiat.*, 1889, 8: 75–115.

19 Neuralgie und Psychose. *Jahrb.Psychiat.*, 1889, 8: 287–292.

20 Julius Wagner-Jauregg. Ueber Osteomalakie und Geistesstörung. *Jahrb.Psychiat.*, 1890, 9: 113–127.

21 Heinrich Obersteiner. Grundzüge einer Geschichte des Vereines für Psychiatrie und Neurologie in Wien in den ersten fünfzig Jahren seines Bestehens (1868–1918). *Jahrb.Psychiat.*, 1919, 39: 1–46.

THREE

GRAZ 1889–93

Wagner-Jauregg moved to Graz in the autumn of 1889. Graz, the ancient capital of Styria and the second largest city in Austria, is beautifully situated on both banks of the river Mur, and enclosed on three sides by wooded heights. Although the University of Graz had an ancient history – it was founded in the sixteenth century – it was closed in 1782 and replaced by a different type of school, the Lyceum, to which was attached a new medicosurgical school. In 1827 the University reopened, but without a medical faculty. Medical teaching remained with the Lyceum until 1863 when the university's own medical faculty was founded and the university turned into a full university.

In 1847 Franz Köstl (1811–82), the medical superintendent at the Graz Asylum, received permission to hold clinical lectures in psychiatry. However, he left the Asylum in 1852 to take up another post and the medical establishment lost its lecturer in the subject. His successor, Donat Land (d. 1872), did not get permission to continue these lectures until 1855. Even then he had difficulty in using patients at the Asylum for demonstrations. In 1867 it was decided to move the Asylum to Feldhof, a location about one hour's journey from Graz. Johann Czermak (1828–73), the director of the Asylum at Brno which was considered as a model, was called to Graz to oversee the project and his proposals were accepted by the Provincial Council in October 1869. Donat Lang was retiring and Czermak took over as Director. However, he died in 1872 and Köstl, at one time the Director, took over in an interim capacity and was responsible for the transfer of the inmates from the new to the old

43

Asylum. Krafft-Ebing took over as Director of the Asylum and was appointed Extraordinary Professor in 1873. Theoretical and practical tuition in psychiatry for medical graduates was approved by the Ministry of Education and the Provincial Council.

When Wagner-Jauregg took over the Graz Clinic conditions there were very different from those in Vienna. In the Vienna Clinic there were a relatively large number of beds, about 150, but also a very small rate of intake of new patients, also about 150 a year, so that the total only renewed itself annually. In Graz the number of psychiatric beds was much smaller, but there was a much greater rate of change of patients because all new admissions came to the Clinic and only a few were sent direct to the Asylum at Feldhof. That meant that Wagner-Jauregg was unable to observe particular patients during the total time of their illness, and never for many years, because he had to find room for new admissions. However, this situation had advantages. It was necessary to make a quick diagnosis of each case, and the large number of cases widened his clinical experience.

The Psychiatric Clinic was combined with a Neurology Clinic which had only between 24 and 30 beds. The wards for psychiatric male patients were very unsatisfactory, having been the stables of the Commandant of the local fortress. One day when Wagner-Jauregg came to visit the ward he saw to his surprise that a board had been lifted from the floor and below there was a channel that ran right through the ward. He discovered that this was the drain for the whole building which in the upper stories contained the obstetric clinic. After he complained, appropriate action was taken to remedy the situation.

At first Wagner-Jauregg did not have enough assistance. Krafft-Ebing had left one assistant behind who, although intelligent and good natured, was very eccentric. After a year he went back to his home in the Tirol and joined the state sanitary service. Another assistant, a Czech, whom Wagner-Jauregg had brought with him from Vienna, did not feel happy in Graz and after half a year went back to Prague to take up veterinary medicine.

Wagner-Jauregg's appointment to the University of Graz had come too late in the year for his lectures to be included in the lecture list for 1889/90, but he began to lecture in the summer semester of 1890. There were about seven or eight students present, including Friedrich Schlagenhaufer (1866–1930) who many years later collaborated with Wagner-Jauregg in his work on cretinism. However,

in his later years in Graz Wagner-Jauregg's lectures were well attended, and he also had the right to hold lectures at the provincial
Asylum of Feldhof, which was under the provincial council of Styria.
He used this opportunity to bring his students two or three times
during a semester in buses to the Asylum where he was able to
present patients during his lecture. These outings were very popular
with the students; they were a kind of excursion which for most
ended with a visit to the nearby brewery, Puntigam.

Wagner-Jauregg, like his predecessor Krafft-Ebing, was not
only Extraordinary Professor but also the chief medical officer of the
General Hospital which was under the provincial council. He therefore not only received a salary from the University but also from the
Province. In addition, he had his private practice, the income from
which nearly doubled during his time at Graz, so that his financial
situation seems to have been very satisfactory. He regularly attended
the weekly meetings of the Medical Society of Styria through which
he came into contact with his colleagues, some of whom gathered
together after the meetings for an evening meal at the principal hotel
in Graz. He was among the more sociable who afterwards went to a
wine bar. He does not say in his *Memoirs* whether he was among the
most indefatigable colleagues who finished the night in a coffee-
house.

As Extraordinary Professor, Wagner-Jauregg was not at first
a member of the professorial board because, according to regulations,
the number of extraordinary professors on the board could be no
more than half the number of ordinary professors. Although Wagner-
Jauregg was the Director of the Clinic, there were extraordinary
professors who were senior to him. However, from the second of his
four years in Graz he became a member of the board with a short
interruption due to the number of ordinary professors having diminished owing to a vacancy.

In 1892/93 he was responsible for a petition to the professorial
board, supported by the paediatrician Theodor Escherich (1857–
1911) and the dermatologist Eduard Lipp (1831–1891), which was
to be submitted to the Ministry of Education by the then Dean of the
Graz Medical Faculty, the ophthalmologist Isidor Schnabel (1842–
1908), advocating a change in the examination regulations with a
view to including paediatrics, psychiatry and dermatology in the
syllabus for the medical diploma. It was argued that anyone who
was entitled to practise medicine was under an obligation to treat
any illness and it was the duty of the State to ensure that the

doctor's knowledge covered the whole range of medicine. The medical curriculum ignored extensive fields of practical medicine, yet the progress of the medical student might be delayed if he did not know the name of some unimportant plant! (Botany was then a part of the curriculum.) The syllabus failed to take proper account of those three important parts of internal medicine which had branched off into separate disciplines. They required special methods of examination and treatment, and the person afflicted by a skin disease or syphilis, the sick child or the mentally ill could find no place in a clinic for internal diseases. No professor of internal medicine could master these branches, even if he had the will to do so, because of the lack of opportunity to see patients suffering from these illnesses. The educational authorities had found it necessary to establish clinics and engage teachers for those disciplines, but although medical students had the opportunity to study them, they were under no obligation to do so.

The petition urged that consideration be given to a far-reaching reform of the medical curriculum, introducing the three disciplines and possibly reducing the less important subjects such as botany, zoology and mineralogy. Pending this major reform, it was suggested that a temporary solution might be for co-examiners to be appointed for those subjects which were not compulsory. The petition urged the professorial board to sponsor an application to the Ministry of Education to consider the proposed reform and to appoint co-examiners for the three disciplines. Thus it was from Graz that the campaign for the revision of the medical syllabus was initiated, but it took several years before the reform materialised.

The Medical Society of Styria had a library in which there were some medical periodicals and a small number of books. Wagner-Jauregg wondered later, when he was able to make use of the excellent library of the Vienna Medical Society after his return there, how he had managed with the meagre resources at Graz. This made scientific work very difficult for him because on the one hand there was no literature to stimulate him and on the other it was difficult to check one's own findings and ideas with those of others. Above all there was no foreign literature. It is not surprising therefore that it was not until the end of 1891 that a paper by him was published in one of the Vienna medical weeklies.[1] This was based on an observation which arose from an earlier publication,[2] dating from his time in Vienna, on the spasms occurring as a result of resuscitating those who had attempted suicide by hanging. In the original paper Wagner-Jauregg considered a number of such cases, some reported in the literature and some based on his own experience, in which the symptoms following resuscitation had been observed. The two main effects were convulsions, which usually occurred after breathing was restored, described by some as of an epileptic or tetanic character, and the lack of memory. He attributed both these symptoms to the damaging effect of asphyxia and the consequent lack of oxygen supply to the brain and/or to the closing of the carotid artery. Retroactive amnesia was described in eleven out of seventeen cases, its degree depending on the duration of suspension and unconsciousness. On the other hand, Wagner-Jauregg found that the attempted suicide seemed to have had a beneficial effect on the mentally sick. He quoted two cases reported in the literature of women suffering from melancholia, one of whom was completely cured, the other showing a temporary improvement. A case he experienced himself concerned a woman of a melancholic and somewhat paranoid nature who had attempted to commit suicide by hanging but was cut down. She suffered from convulsions and amnesia after the attempt, but was subsequently cured of her mental illness.

The case that provoked the 1891 paper was one that came before the Graz County Court in which, as a result of a fight, a son had severely injured his father and then tried to hang himself. He was discovered and cut down. He suffered from the two symptoms described in the earlier paper, namely convulsions and amnesia, and the man's memory returned several days later. Wagner-Jauregg believed that amnesia following asphyxia was similar to that occurring after concussion or an epileptic fit, all being due to circulatory disturbances.

These two papers involved Wagner-Jauregg in a controversy with the German neurologist P.J. Moebius (1853–1907), who claimed in an article in a Munich medical weekly that at least in some cases the symptoms described by Wagner-Jauregg were due to traumatic hysteria.[3] Not only the convulsions but also the amnesia were a consequence of the emotional upset. Since amnesia occurred not only after hanging but also after suicide attempts by shooting, the reason must be the emotional disturbance which prevented memories from entering consciousness. He quoted a case recorded by Charcot in which memory returned under hypnosis. Wagner-Jauregg replied in an article, published in the same periodical a year later,[4] in which he adhered to his point of view, insisting that the convulsions were not of a hysterical nature. Proof of this was that they had also been observed in cats and dogs which had been strangled, and he referred to animal experiments with cats and rabbits which he had performed himself. Moebius in his reply[5] adhered to his thesis, claiming that factors leading to suicide were of a nature that would be likely to lead to hysteria. If the symptoms were purely physiological, why did they not occur after strokes and brain haemorrhage. In his *Memoirs*, written over forty years after the publication of these articles, Wagner-Jauregg speaks of Moebius having referred to him in a very unscientific fashion and 'having attacked him, adopting a very superior tone'.[6] On reading these articles and the two final papers published during the same year it is difficult to understand why Wagner-Jauregg seems to have got so upset by the controversy. The only personal remark made by Moebius is one in which he refers to Wagner-Jauregg as being one of those psychiatrists who had great enthusiasm for the anatomic-physiologic point of view and sought to explain everything physiologically. That was why Wagner-Jauregg rejected his arguments and wanted to know nothing of hysteria. In his final reply to Moebius[7] Wagner-Jauregg said that he only knew two methods of scientific research: observation and experiment.

An important paper which he wrote during the same period was on the subject of 'Somatic bases of acute psychoses'.[8] It arose from a request to address an out-of-town meeting in Graz of the Society for Psychiatry and Neurology in Vienna in October 1891. The lecture was a great success and Meynert could not forbear to combine his appreciation of it with a spiteful remark against his old dead enemy Leidesdorf by calling Wagner-Jauregg a famous autodidact. In it Wagner-Jauregg claimed that, although mental illness had been recognised as brain disease, and brain anatomy and physiology were the bases for the study of mental disturbances, it was necessary to go back to the processes which caused these by appealing to the whole field of clinical medicine for their understanding. As an analogy he quoted jaundice, which was not, as might be thought, a skin disease. It was possible that mental sickness was not necessarily caused by brain disease, but by the disease of some other organ, for example the intestinal canal, which caused the healthy brain to function abnormally. Metabolic products of bacteria can have a toxic effect on the nervous system, and gastrointestinal disturbances can be followed by psychoses. The analysis of the urine in mental patients sometimes shows the presence of toxic substances, e.g. acetone or albumen.

In 1892 Wagner-Jauregg published a paper 'On the squeez-able bladder'.[9] This was the result of an investigation carried out over some time on the innervation of the bladder. In cases of a paralysed bladder as a result of spinal cord disease it was found that, if pressure was brought to bear on the abdomen, it was often possible to cause the urine to flow away. Wagner-Jauregg tried to find out what made this possible, concluding that, in cases of atonic paralysis of the bladder, it was effectively squeezable, but not so in cases of tonic paralysis. He did not pursue the subject himself, but it stimulated Lothar von Frankl-Hochwart (1862–1914) to make ex-periments on animals. During the same year and during 1892/93 Wagner-Jauregg worked on a number of articles on psychiatry for a medical encyclopaedia.[10] He wrote on mania, melancholia, dementia paralytica, idiocy and hysteria – altogether sixty pages.

In 1892 Wagner-Jauregg also resumed research which he had begun in 1884 with his animal experiments on the removal of the thyroid gland, now approaching the problem from a different angle. What led him to take it up again was the arrival from Innsbruck of an old friend from his student days, Moriz Holl, who had been appointed professor of anatomy at Graz about the time Wagner-Jauregg came there. They often went on excursions into the moun-tains together, and Holl was greatly disturbed by the number of cretins they met. He impressed on Wagner-Jauregg that as a psy-chiatrist he ought to investigate the problems of cretinism. Wagner-Jauregg took up the challenge and for very many years devoted much time and work to the study of this important question. This will be told in a later chapter.

Wagner-Jauregg liked living in Graz and got much pleasure from the surrounding countryside and his walks in the mountains. He made a large circle of friends and in September 1890, a year after he took up his duties, he was married to Balbine Frumkin, née Goldberg, whose first marriage was dissolved in Warsaw in March of that year. From personal reminiscences by Helene Deutsch, related by Paul Roazen,[11] it appears that Balbine had been a patient of his whom he treated for morphine addiction. He married her, convinced that she had been cured. Balbine had two children from her first marriage, a son Jakob and a daughter Melanie, born in 1882, to whom Wagner-Jauregg became very attached. In his *Memoirs* he never speaks of his private life and there is only one mention of his wife and step-daughter in connection with a holiday in the environs of Graz. One of the witnesses to the marriage was his colleague Theodor Escherich, with whose family he must have been on very friendly terms. Among his archives there is some correspondence with Theodor Escherich's daughter, Sonya Weber, who addresses him as 'Uncle Julius'.

Wagner-Jauregg's years in Graz seem to have been a very happy period of his life. When, therefore, in 1892 the post of Director at the First Psychiatric Clinic in Vienna (a far more prestigious post than the one in Graz) became vacant after Krafft-Ebing had moved to the Second Psychiatric Clinic at the General Hospital following Meynert's death in 1892, the possibility that the First Clinic might be discontinued did not unduly disappoint him. He thought that it would be considered superfluous, particularly since psychiatry was still not a compulsory subject in the medical syllabus, and he was content to remain in Graz.

However, things turned out differently. The authorities decided to continue the First Psychiatric Clinic at the Asylum, and to make a new appointment. Three candidates had been short-listed, two of whom were very distinguished psychiatrists, Eduard Hitzig (1838–1907) and Carl Wernicke (1848–1905). It so happened that in the spring of 1893 Wagner-Jauregg was in Vienna for his brother's wedding and happened to run into a friend (in his old age Wagner-Jauregg could not remember whether it was Stricker's nephew or his former Colleague Dr Gärtner), who told him to go and see Stricker who wanted to speak to him. Wagner-Jauregg explained that he had deliberately not visited him because he felt that it might have looked as if he wanted Stricker to intercede on his behalf in the appointment of Krafft-Ebing's successor. However, he went to see him and at Stricker's request called on Krafft-Ebing. It was purely a courtesy visit and nothing was said about the pending appointment.

When the subject came up at the meeting of the professorial board, Stricker suggested that Wagner-Jauregg's name be added to the list of candidates. Krafft-Ebing, who had to report on the appointment, agreed and several professors supported the proposal. Nevertheless, Wagner-Jauregg did not think that he had much hope of getting the post because Hitzig and Wernicke were far more distinguished. However, both refused the offer of appointment, which left only two candidates, Arnold Pick (1851–1924) and himself. Wagner-Jauregg was not particularly keen on moving to Vienna, yet he was clearly anxious for the promotion. At one time he wondered whether to withdraw his application, and he did something which might have seemed crass stupidity but which turned out in his favour. In his *Memoirs* he comments that 'if one is in luck, even stupid actions turn out to one's advantage'.[12] He knew the weakness of the Asylum Clinic from experience: the Professor and Director of the Clinic was under the Director of the Asylum who received his instructions not from the central government but from the provincial government. This had caused difficulties in the past. The disagreements between Meynert, the Professor in charge of the Clinic and Ludwig Schlager (1828–85), the Director of the Asylum were notorious and the relations between Meynert's successor, Leidesdorf, and Schlager were none too happy either. In a section of Wagner-Jauregg's *Memoirs*, not included in the published version, he tells how Schlager insisted that Leidesdorf, as head of the medical staff, reside at the Asylum. Leidesdorf, who had a beautiful home in the outskirts of Vienna, had no intention of doing so. Schlager allocated to him a room at the Asylum for which he had to pay rent. It was the smallest room in the place and Leidesdorf never set foot in it.

In the circumstances, it is not surprising that Wagner-Jauregg decided to travel to Vienna to see Dr Weitlof who was in charge of the department responsible for the provincial hospitals. Wagner-Jauregg told him that his name had been put forward as a possible head of the Psychiatric Clinic at the Asylum, but explained that he would not accept the post, if it was offered to him, unless he was assured that, when the post of Director of the Asylum became vacant, he would obtain that appointment, too, in addition to his post at the Clinic. He knew all about the disagreements which had occurred between the Head of the Clinic and the Director of the Asylum who was his superior.

Not only did Weitlof agree to his request, but he wrote to the Ministry of Education to say that the provincial government was prepared to transfer the responsibility of directing the Asylum to the Head of the Clinic if Wagner-Jauregg was appointed. This seemed to have been the decisive step in assuring Wagner-Jauregg's appointment to the post. The Minister knew full well of the frequent conflicts between the Clinic and the Director of the Asylum and thought that these conflicts would be avoided if the two posts were held by the same person.

In Graz Wagner-Jauregg was Extraordinary Professor, which was the general rule in the subject of psychiatry. Leidesdorf had been an extraordinary professor, as were Meynert and Krafft-Ebing at first. They were given personal chairs relatively late in their careers when they threatened to accept posts abroad. Wagner-Jauregg therefore expected to be appointed Extraordinary Professor in Vienna, but during the last days of September 1893 he received a telegram from his father congratulating him on his appointment to a chair. He could scarcely believe this and thought at first that his father must have been misinformed. However, a few days later he got the letter confirming his appointment, which was of immense importance to him because it brought with it membership of the professorial board.

REFERENCES

1 Julius Wagner-Jauregg. Ueber einige Erscheinungen im Bereiche des Centralnervensystems, welche nach Wiederbelebung Erhängter beobachtet werden. *Jahrb.Psychiat.*, 1889, 8: 313–332.

2 Julius Wagner-Jauregg. Psychische Störungen nach Wiederbelebung eines Erhängten. *Wien.Klin.Wschr.*, 1891, 4: no. 53, 998–1002.

3 P.J. Moebius. Ueber die Seelenstörungen nach Selbstmordversuchen. *Münch.Med.Wschr.*, 1892, 39: no. 36, 631–633.

4 Julius Wagner-Jauregg. Ueber Krämpfe und Amnesie nach Wiederbelebung Erhängter. *Münch.Med.Wschr.*, 1893, 40: no. 5, 87–91.

5 P.J. Moebius. Bemerkungen zu dem Aufsatz Prof. Wagners 'Ueber Krämpfe und Amnesie nach Wiederbelebung Erhängter.' *Münch.Med.Wschr.*, 1893, 40: no. 7, 127–129.

6 Julius Wagner-Jauregg. *Lebenserinnerungen.* Ed. L. Schönbauer und M. Jantsch. Wien: Springer Verlag, 1950, p. 52.

7 Julius Wagner-Jauregg. Noch ein Wort über Krämpfe und Amnesie nach Wiederbelebung Erhängter. Eine Erwiderung an P.J. Moebius. *Münch.Med.Wschr.*, 1893, 40: no. 10, 194.

8 Julius Wagner-Jauregg. Ueber die körperlichen Grundlagen der acuten Psychosen. *Jahrb.Psychiat.*, 1891, 10: 180–198.

9 Julius Wagner-Jauregg. Ueber die ausdruckbare Blase. Beitrag zur Kenntnis der Innervationsstörungen der Blase. *Wien.Klin. Wschr.*, 1892, 5: no. 47, 671–674.

10 *Bibliothek der gesamten medizinischen Wissenschaften für praktische Aerzte und Specialaerzte.* Wien und Leipzig: M. Merlin, 1893–1896.

[11] Paul Roazen. *Helene Deutsch. A Psychoanalyst's Life.* New American Library, 1985.

[12] Wagner-Jauregg, op.cit. ref 6, p. 54.

FOUR

Return to Vienna

The First Psychiatric Clinic

The beginnings of psychiatry in Austria date back to the period of the Enlightenment. Shortly after the Emperor Joseph II succeeded to the throne in 1780 he decided that the General Hospital then under construction was to include a building for the keeping and treatment of insane persons. This came to be known as the 'Narrenturm' (Fools' Tower) which still exists as a Museum, but even now it looks gloomy and menacing. It contained 139 securely barred cells on five floors, where the insane were protected from self-inflicted harm by means of iron chains which also served to shield those around them against attacks. By order of the Emperor, the insane were taken outside for a walk whenever possible, and instructions for the staff, published in 1789, strictly forbade cruel treatment of the mentally ill. Patients were accepted in the Narrenturm until 1869, but in 1853 a new asylum was opened and gradually the no-restraint-system, pioneered in England, was introduced in the new institution.[1]

Already towards the end of the eighteenth century many specialist clinics had been set up in Vienna, but it was some time before the First Psychiatric Clinic was inaugurated. When the asylums were transferred from central to provincial government control, the central government reserved the right to institute a psychiatric clinic at the Vienna Asylum. This was at the suggestion of Max Leidesdorf. The right was exercised in 1870, and the First Psychiatric Clinic in Austria was founded at the Vienna Asylum (the Asylum for Lower Austria) as the result of a decree dated 1 July 1870. Three candidates hoped to be appointed as Director. They were Max Leidesdorf, the Director of the private asylum at Döbling (on the outskirts of Vienna); Theodor Meynert, Privatdozent and Prosector at the Vienna Asylum; and Ludwig Schlager, the Extraordinary Professor of Psychiatry, who was in charge of the department of observation of mental conditions with uncertain diagnosis at the General Hospital.

The decision lay in the hands of Carl von Rokitansky, the well-known pathological anatomist, consultant to the Ministry of Education and the most important medical authority in the country. In the event Meynert was appointed to the post, and an agreement concerning finance, administration and service between the Council responsible for the Asylum and the Ministry responsible for the Clinic was signed in November 1870. According to A. Pilcz (1871–1954),[2] owing to the understanding of the Council and the personal character of the Director of the Asylum no conflict arose between the teaching needs of the Clinic and the administrative requirements of the Asylum.

That this was not always the case is shown by the events that occurred about three years after Meynert's appointment, events not only commented on in the contemporary medical literature[3] of Vienna but also by Wagner-Jauregg[4] in an article on the history of the psychiatric clinics published in 1936, and by E. Lesky.[5] The trouble seems to have begun with the appointment of Professor Ludwig Schlager as Director of the Asylum. Since the Clinic which Meynert directed was a department of the Asylum, he and Schlager were now brought into close contact. Unfortunately, they had not seen eye to eye with one another for some time: indeed, as representatives of University and Asylum psychiatry they were in opposing camps. Furthermore, Schlager believed that his efforts to reform Austrian mental health regulations were being undermined by Meynert's neuroanatomical research. There were also administrative difficulties which, together with the other problems, led to their relationship becoming so strained that the Provincial Council forced Meynert's resignation.

However, Rokitansky continued to support Meynert and in 1875 created out of the department of observation at the General Hospital a second psychiatric clinic with Meynert as its Director. Leidesdorf, who had been head of that department since Schlager became Director of the Asylum, was appointed to the post vacated by Meynert and made Extraordinary Professor. Thus, although psychiatry was not a compulsory subject and did not form part of the medical syllabus – it was made an obligatory subject only in 1903 –

the Vienna medical faculty became unique in having two psychiatric clinics.

The affair was commented on widely in the local medical press, which described it as a 'psychiatric coup d'état'.[6] It was obvious that the new Clinic had been created so as to provide a post for Meynert. The writer of an article in one of the Vienna medical weeklies[7] argued that to convert the department of observation into a clinic was not in the interests of the General Hospital. The purpose of the department of observation was to deal with cases of mental disturbance with uncertain diagnoses, which included patients from other departments of the hospital. The maximum stay of patients was fourteen days, so that with 67 beds available more than a thousand patients might pass through the department annually. To turn a department with such a rapid turnover of patients into a clinic would require patients to stay for eight to twelve weeks, so that the whole course of the disease and the result of the treatment might be observed.

At that time only about twelve students, mostly graduates, were allowed to attend lectures during which patients were demonstrated. The writer of the article argued that it would be objectionable to exhibit patients during lectures to the larger audience of students that would attend a university clinic. He claimed that changing a short-stay psychiatric department into a psychiatric clinic would destroy a humanitarian service without improving teaching. He also took a poor view of Meynert, whom he accused of lacking any enthusiasm for the subject of psychiatry.

Despite the opposition in the medical press, Meynert's appointment was confirmed, and in 1887 he even succeeded in persuading the authorities to add a neurological clinic to his psychiatric clinic at the General Hospital by threatening to accept an appointment elsewhere. In 1889 Leidesdorf, the Director of the First Psychiatric Clinic, died and was succeeded by Richard von Krafft-Ebing, who had been Professor and Director of the psychiatric clinic at Graz. He in turn took over Meynert's post after the latter's death in 1892. He, like Meynert, did not feel happy at the First Psychiatric Clinic at the Asylum, whose Director, Moriz Gauster (1828–95), was responsible to the government of Lower Austria and had no academic post. So when Meynert died, Krafft-Ebing was glad to be appointed to succeed him. Thus, the position of Director of the First Psychiatric Clinic became vacant. As already mentioned, Wagner-Jauregg did not think that the Clinic would be continued since it seemed superfluous, particularly as psychiatry was still not part of the medical syllabus. Nevertheless, it was decided to continue the Clinic and Wagner-Jauregg was chosen as the new Director.

In his history of the First Psychiatric Clinic Pilcz[8] emphasised the great advantage it possessed compared with other University Institutions. These stemmed particularly from the Clinic being part of an Asylum and the fact that the patients were very different, both in practical as well as in clinical respects, from those encountered in other psychiatric clinics. Many details of the practical care of the insane, also the final outcome of the many forms of psychoses and the whole course of mental disturbances could only be studied in an asylum. On the other hand, many of the short-lived mental disturbances, febrile deliriums and acute functional psychoses rarely reached the Asylum. Individuals who were suspected by the police doctor of being mentally disturbed could not, according to statute, be admitted direct to the Asylum, but had to be sent for observation to the Second Psychiatric Clinic at the General Hospital. Moreover, although the Clinic had an outpatient department for nervous diseases, it could not admit patients suffering from these.

Krafft-Ebing, Wagner-Jauregg's predecessor, writing about the Vienna Psychiatric Clinics in 1890,[9] claimed that the First Clinic performed the functions of a hospital department and was not really suitable for instructing medical students. The number of patients admitted annually to the Asylum was very large and the number of beds in the Clinic alone was 200. Of those barely 40 might be suitable for purposes of instruction. Admissions took place in such a way that only every third patient was sent to the Clinic and the Clinic had no right to keep cases of clinical interest and send the others to the Asylum. One of Wagner-Jauregg's assistants, E. Stransky, in his *Memoirs*[10] called it the 'Cinderella' Clinic.

Wagner-Jauregg at the First Clinic

When Wagner-Jauregg returned to the Clinic where he had been assistant, he found conditions much as they had been when he had left for Graz. The Asylum was under the direction of Moriz Gauster, who was a friend of his and his family and with whom he got on very well. As for assistance, he was in a better position than he had been in Graz. When Krafft-Ebing left Graz for Vienna he took with him two assistants, Dr Kasparek whom Wagner-Jauregg clearly disliked (he calls him a man of little worth)[11] and with whom he had had unpleasant encounters, both professionally and personally; and Ernst Boeck (1857–1924). On his transfer to the Clinic at the General Hospital, the Second Psychiatric Clinic, Krafft-Ebing took Dr Kasparek with him, but Boeck, who had not got on particularly well with his chief, preferred to remain at the Clinic at the Asylum and become Wagner-Jauregg's assistant. Wagner-Jauregg liked him and found him an engaging personality and very well read. He was of a similar age and had an impressive presence, with 'a beautiful full beard' according to Wagner-Jauregg.[12] Quite often people who came to the Clinic turned to Boeck, thinking he was the professor. At Wagner-Jauregg's suggestion, Boeck carried out experiments with tuberculin to test the curative effect of feverish infectious diseases on insanity, experiments which Wagner-Jauregg had already begun at the Graz Clinic. A detailed account of these is given in the chapter on fever therapy. Boeck remained at the Clinic until his appointment as Chief Medical Officer at the Silesian Asylum at Troppau in 1895.

As his other assistant Wagner-Jauregg chose Dr J. Starlinger, who was assistant physician at the Asylum, but who wanted to carry out some brain research. As Starlinger was not experienced in animal experiments Wagner-Jauregg assisted him with these, the object of which was to observe the effect of cutting through the nerves in the pyramidal tract of the extended spinal column. According to the theory then prevailing on the function of these nerves, cutting through them would result in paralysing all four extremities of the animal. However, Wagner-Jauregg had already conducted such an experiment on a dog when he was working at Stricker's Laboratory. As expected, the animal seemed quite paralysed after the operation, but then something strange happened. Stricker kept a violin at the Laboratory and was wont to pick it up occasionally and play a tune. He did so on this occasion, whereupon the dog rose on all four legs and followed Stricker around.

It was Wagner-Jauregg's intention to carry out the operation in such a way that the animal would keep alive for some time to allow the wound to heal. Wagner-Jauregg describes in some detail how he performed this very difficult operation on a number of dogs, a procedure which, he claims, has never been repeated by anyone else. The result was that the animals recovered and were able to walk and jump about as usual. Wagner-Jauregg let Starlinger publish the discovery of the extrapyramidal tract which he presented to the Society for Psychiatry in Vienna at a meeting of 12 February

1895.[13] Freud, who was in the audience, expressed his astonishment at the unexpected results of the experiments. As Wagner-Jauregg comments in his *Memoirs* 'at that time Freud was still more of a neurologist than a psychoanalyst.'[14]

From the entries in the Calendar for the University of Vienna it appears that Emil Redlich (1866–1930) and Adolf Elzholz (1863–1925) succeeded Boeck and Starlinger as Wagner-Jauregg's assistants in the latter part of 1895. Redlich had been working in Heinrich Obersteiner's Laboratory and had produced some interesting papers, including one on the posterior roots of the spinal cord and the well-known Obersteiner-Redlich theory of the origin of tabes. Strangely, Wagner-Jauregg says in his *Memoirs* that he succeeded in persuading Redlich that his theory was wrong![15] Redlich was very useful to Wagner-Jauregg because he kept abreast of recent developments in psychiatry and was able to draw the attention of his chief to them. Wagner-Jauregg had little time for reading anything that was not of immediate concern, which is not surprising in view of his many duties and interests. Redlich specialised in the pathology and aetiology of epilepsy, a subject on which he wrote extensively. Wagner-Jauregg calls him a good assistant because he upheld his own opinions and convictions and would only change his mind if he was convinced of the rightness of the argument, not because of pressure by his superior. According to Wagner-Jauregg the bad assistants are those who were good only at auscultation and, whether in diagnosis or scientific work, followed the opinions of their superior.

Elzholz had been recommended to Wagner-Jauregg by Edmund von Neusser who became an assistant in Bamberger's Clinic at the time Wagner-Jauregg hoped to be appointed. Neusser had become ordinary professor in the same year as his one-time competitor. Elzholz had worked under Neusser at one of the Vienna hospitals, but failed to get an assistantship at Neusser's Clinic. However, Neusser had promised him that, if he took up psychiatry, he would support him if and when the chair of psychiatry at Cracow or Lvov became vacant, Neusser having considerable influence in Polish circles. Elzholz therefore joined Wagner-Jauregg's team and did much good work, eventually being appointed a University Lecturer and remaining with Wagner-Jauregg during all his years at the First Psychiatric Clinic. However, when a vacancy did occur at Lvov University, Elzholz was not chosen because he was a Jew and refused to be baptised. Soon after, he left the Clinic and accepted a post as psychiatric consultant to the Supreme Court in Vienna, but the disappointment he suffered probably caused him to give up all scientific work. He never published another paper.

In 1899 Emil Redlich, whose assistance Wagner-Jauregg had greatly appreciated and whom he regarded as a friend, left the Clinic. Two new assistants, A. Pilcz and E. Raimann (1872–1949), joined the staff.

In 1895 the Director of the Asylum, Moriz Gauster, had died. As will be remembered, Wagner-Jauregg, when applying for the post at the First Psychiatric Clinic, had stipulated that he would only accept the post of Director if, in the event that the directorship of the Asylum became vacant, he would be appointed to that post. However, there were two reasons which persuaded him not to insist on his demand being met. First, Lueger's Christian Socialist Party* had made such progress that it was to be expected that it would seize control of the Provincial Council, and Wagner-Jauregg did not relish the idea of having a member of that party as his chief. He discussed the matter with his friend at the Ministry, Dr Weitlof, who advised him not to accept the post of Director. The second reason was an event that he foresaw although it did not happen for some years. Because the Asylum was becoming too small, it had been suggested that, instead of extending the building on its present site, it would be better to sell it with the freehold and to build a larger and more modern asylum with the proceeds at some distance from the city. Although Wagner-Jauregg agreed with this suggestion in principle, he realised that if he became Director he would have to move out of the city, and this would put an end to his clinical activites. He therefore did not object to the appointment of Adalbert Tilkovsky (1871–1907), who had been a colleague when he first came to the Asylum.

WAGNER-JAUREGG'S LECTURES

Wagner-Jauregg did not begin his regular courses of lectures until the summer semester of 1894, but he gave his inaugural lecture[16] on taking up his Chair and the directorship of the First Psychiatric Clinic in 1893. In it he spoke on the teaching of psychiatry and the relation of the subject with the anatomy and physiology of the brain,

---

* Karl Lueger (1844–1910).

and with neuropathology and forensic medicine. He described the work of his predecessors in the Chair: Leidesdorf, Meynert and Krafft-Ebing. But the main theme of his address was the importance of the misuse of alcohol and of heredity in the aetiology of mental diseases. In his view – and in this he was clearly much influenced by the ideas of Benedict Morel (1809–73) – degeneration played an important part and degenerates often ended up in asylums or in prisons. He referred to Lombroso's idea* that criminals show physical and psychological characteristics which mark them out as a special anthropological type of the human race.

Wagner-Jauregg's first course of lectures in the summer semester of 1894 was on 'Special pathology, therapy and clinical aspects of psychiatric diseases'.[17] He lectured three times a week from 5–6.30 p.m. He repeated this course in the next three semesters, but in the winter semester of 1895/96 he also lectured three times a week from 12–1 p.m. on 'Special pathology, therapy and clinical aspects of nervous diseases'. He did so again during the winter semester of 1896/97, but during the following years he gave only the psychiatry lectures, which he continued until he moved to the Second Psychiatric Clinic at the General Hospital in 1902. In later years he lectured mostly on nervous diseases and held practical sessions on psychiatry.

When Stransky, who later became his assistant, was a medical student at the University, he was most impressed by the lectures on psychiatry.[18] It was by chance that he opted to attend those by Wagner-Jauregg rather than those by Krafft-Ebing whose sensationally mounted lectures were attended not only by undergraduates but also by laymen, particularly journalists. He described Wagner-Jauregg's lectures as rather dry, suggesting sometimes a certain boredom, but the demonstrations of mentally ill patients were fascinating, although not presented in the sensational way used by Krafft-Ebing whose lectures were more like theatrical performances than clinical lectures.

In an appreciation of Wagner-Jauregg on the occasion of his 75th birthday the neurologist I.P. Karplus tells how, when he had been made head of the neurology department at the General Hospital and was anxious to revise his psychiatric knowledge, he attended Wagner-Jauregg's lectures during a winter semester.[19] He

---

* Cesare Lombroso (1835–1909).

speaks of his outstanding clinical lectures and his masterly art of exposition. Wagner-Jauregg tried to explain mental phenomena from psychological principles and physiological matters purely from physiology, thus avoiding the fault of so many psychiatrists in their lectures by jumping from one subject to another. He would analyse a case so as to give the impression of a convincing experiment. In his talk with the patient the facts became clear and their consequences were made explicit to his listeners.

According to F. Hochstetter (1861–1954), Wagner-Jauregg was outstanding and unsurpassed as a teacher.[20] His students spoke of the clarity with which he explained complicated relations and of how stimulating his lectures were. Dr S. Last described Wagner-Jauregg as a very good lecturer who always kept to his subject,[21] maintaining a very modest mien and not taking credit for his achievements.

Wagner-Jauregg' clinical work

In the early days of his career Wagner-Jauregg wanted to become a specialist in internal medicine, and throughout his life he was always looking for the somatic origin of nervous and psychiatric diseases. As Otto Pötzl (1877–1962) wrote in his Obituary,[22] he was the first to introduce into psychiatry the thought-processes of internal medicine. His two great achievements, the malaria therapy of GPI and the thyroidal theory of cretinism basically dealt with organic diseases, GPI being a late stage of syphilis and cretinism arising from the malfunction of the thyroid.

Already in 1891, in a lecture in Graz,[23] and later in a paper presented in 1896[24] he was outlining his belief that there was not only a relation between infectious illness and polyneuritis, but also between psychoses and gastrointestinal troubles. He wondered whether metabolic products of bacteria might have toxic effects on the nervous system and could cause post-febrile psychoses. Wagner-Jauregg complained in his *Memoirs*[25] that this paper had never been sufficiently appreciated. According to Paul Roazen[26], Helene Deutsch, who worked as an assistant at the Clinic during the First World War, recalled how Wagner-Jauregg put great emphasis on constitution in cases of depression; since it was important for such patients to have their bowel movements, he would enquire whether they had had their enemas. This was an example of his good clinical insight and his acute powers of observation which led him to realise how depression could be a body problem. In later years he encouraged his assistant Raimann to carry out important work on carbohydrate metabolism and the change in the assimilation limit for dextrose in those suffering from melancholia.

According to Pötzl,[27] his successor at the Psychiatric Clinic, Wagner-Jauregg's views at the beginning of his teaching career coincided with those in the early editions of Kraepelin's textbooks* (up to 1902), of which he thought highly and which he recommended to his students. His views did not change greatly: he was inclined to consider the two great categories of Kraepelin's psychiatry, dementia praecox and manic-depressive psychoses, as naturally related groups, rather than as separate units of disease. He rejected changes in nomenclature, even when they had become accepted. 'The facts remain the same; only the names change', he often said, when such problems were discussed.

Wagner-Jauregg was against the separation of 'endogenous' and 'exogenous' psychoses, i.e. a division between inherited diseases and those that were reactions to environmental factors. Pötzl remarks that it is not surprising that the founder of an effective therapy for psychoses should adopt the view that 'with the increase in our knowledge of the pathology of psychoses they will probably be considered more as exogenous'. Wagner-Jauregg adhered to the fundamental concept of acute psychosis, particularly as regards melancholia and conditions of acute hallucinatory confusion (termed 'amentia' by Meynert). Melancholia, when it affected hormonal and metabolic processes, was for him a disease in its own right, without reference to its future periodicity.

Wagner-Jauregg impressed on his students that to understand and treat mentally disturbed and neurotic patients, it was necessary to be familiar with the results of psychology such as are experienced in medical practice at the bedside and in the surgery. That is why he rejected in the treatment of the sick a psychology based on philosophical considerations. He appreciated intuitive sensitivity, but rejected everything of a speculative nature. He was much occupied with practical psychology, particularly social therapy for asocial and antisocial individuals.

Helene Deutsch described her chief as a sensitive psychiatrist and very human.[28] He was as much a clinician as a scientist. He

---

*Emil Kraepelin (1856–1926).

was very good-hearted and concerned about his patients. On ward rounds he remembered which patient was suffering most acutely and he went to that one first. He had a deep, soothing voice that had a great therapeutic effect. His son, in his autobiography[29] speaks of his father's impressive personality and his power of persuasion which often enabled him to cure his patients in a far shorter time than would have been required for psychoanalytic treatment. Stransky also speaks of his personal psychological influence on most patients that was very beneficial, although he might have seemed rather rough to decadent and fussy neuropathic patients. In a lengthy article on Wagner-Jauregg's psychotherapy Stransky claims that, although he was very sceptical of contemporary tendencies in psychiatry, his attitude to psychological methods of treatment was not negative.

As far as addicts and alcoholics were concerned, Wagner-Jauregg's psychotherapeutic tactics were strict and harsh. Nevertheless, he advocated the establishment of institutions for curing alcoholics, but he did all he could not to make them so comfortable in his Clinic that they would consider it a refuge to which they would be glad to return. He therefore isolated relapsed alcoholics in cells and put them on a diet of milk in the belief that this drastic method would induce them to abstain.

Wagner-Jauregg did not think much of beautifying and modernising old-fashioned hospital wards and was against making asylums for drinkers too comfortable. Although he was far from approving the way in which the mentally sick had been treated in the past, he was against spending too much on the incurably mentally ill and asocial, at the expense of the potentially healthy and normal who seemed to him the most precious part of the community. He did not believe that surroundings mattered greatly in the care and treatment of psychotics, and did not object to the use of straitjackets or restraint beds in urgent cases. However, he thought that occupational therapy was beneficial. Wagner-Jauregg recognised the need for psychological treatment of neurotics and Freud's merits in this respect, but he had no liking for the schools of depth psychology and denied them any curative value. Dr S. Last[31] knew of a young woman whom Wagner-Jauregg was treating for severe agoraphobia by making her go out for walks with a companion. He suggested that at first they walked together, then gradually separate, making the distances between them increase just a little each time, clearly anticipating behaviour modification therapy.

Apart from his university lectures and his clinical work, Wagner-Jauregg continued with his scientific investigations into cretinism and the effect of fever therapy on GPI. A number of papers on cretinism belong to this period and an address on fever therapy to the Vienna Medical Society in February 1895. Both these are dealt with in later chapters.

In 1902 Krafft-Ebing retired from his post at the Second Psychiatric Clinic at the General Hospital. By that time Wagner-Jauregg had become firmly established in the medical life of Vienna. He had been appointed a member of the Senior Health Council and had become a prominent figure in the Vienna Medical Society. It is not surprising that he was anxious to succeed Krafft-Ebing, since the Second Clinic was the more prestigious and was associated with a Clinic for Nervous Diseases. Moreover, a project for moving the Asylum out of the centre into the outskirts of Vienna was in the air which would have left Wagner-Jauregg as a Professor of Psychiatry without a Clinic.

However, at first he made no efforts to be considered as the successor, since he did not think it appropriate until Krafft-Ebing's retirement had been finalised. This reticence, according to Wagner-Jauregg's *Memoirs*, nearly cost him the post.[32] Fortunately, he was told by an assistant of Krafft-Ebing, H. von Halban (1870–1926), that Wagner-Jauregg's successor in Graz, Professor Gabriel Anton (1858–1933), would like to move to Vienna and that Krafft-Ebing, who was regretting his resignation which had been tendered in 'dramatic circumstances', was not averse to succeeding Anton at Graz where he had been very happy. The Minister of Education had been told that Wagner-Jauregg was not interested in moving to the General Hospital and preferred to remain at the Asylum. When he heard of this, Wagner-Jauregg lost no time in calling on the Minister to explain why he had not applied before and to ask that his request to succeed Krafft-Ebing be considered. This request was granted and Wagner-Jauregg became Director of the Second Psychiatric Clinic.

No corroboration of this account of the affair has been found. The reference to Krafft-Ebing's request to be retired in dramatic circumstances is puzzling, as is his wish to return to a position in

Graz since he was already a sick man at the time. That Professor
Anton might have wished to move to Vienna is more than likely. In
recounting the incident Wagner-Jauregg sounds somewhat peeved,
but in a speech to commemorate Krafft-Ebing's thirty years' jubilee
as a professor in the same year there is no feeling of resentment.[33]

The work at the Clinic at the General Hospital was very
different from that at the old Clinic at the Asylum where it was
possible to observe the course of a mental illness for years. The
number of beds was similar, about 150, but there were many more
admissions and the change-over of patients was far more rapid.
There was no opportunity to watch individual cases right through,
and there was less intimate contact with the assistants than at the
First Clinic, where the same room served as lecture room, laboratory
and office. The laboratory of the Hospital Clinic was on the second
floor of the Pathological Institute, which was across the road from
the Clinic itself. Wagner-Jauregg realised that in these circumstances
fruitful histological work was not possible without a laboratory assistant. One of Wagner-Jauregg's assistants, E. Raimann, who had
followed him to his new post, suggested his sister-in-law, Klara
Strasky, who was eager to learn. She was trained by Wagner-Jauregg
and his assistants and paid by Wagner-Jauregg out of his own
resources from 1903 until the outbreak of the First World War.
Eventually, he approached the Ministry and convinced them of the
need for such assistance for which he was no longer prepared to pay.
After the war, when the Social Democrats came into power, she was
given a proper status with salary and pension. She was still at the
Clinic, instructing young medical men in their laboratory work,
when Wagner-Jauregg wrote his *Memoirs* and was in his words
'upholding the tradition of the Clinic'.[34]

The Clinic at the General Hospital had one great advantage
over the Clinic at the Asylum in being part of a large hospital and
without the need for the tiresome and time-consuming formalities
necessary for admission to an asylum. Also it had a department
for nervous diseases. Krafft-Ebing, in his article on the Psychiatric
Clinics,[35] claimed that the Second Clinic was not really a Clinic
but a Department for Observation, where the patients were only
incidentally used for instruction. Accommodation was very limited
considering the number of patients.

No one was appointed to succeed Wagner-Jauregg as head of
the First Psychiatric Clinic when he moved to the Second Clinic at
the General Hospital. A. Pilcz, one of Wagner-Jauregg's assistants

remained as Acting Head for five years until the two clinics were combined. Soon after Wagner-Jauregg took over the Second Clinic, negotiations were begun for moving the Asylum from the centre of Vienna to Steinhof in the outskirts. The Government bought the land and with the proceeds the Provincial Council of Lower Austria, which was in charge of the Asylum, erected new prestigious buildings. The architect was Otto Wagner. The complex of buildings includes sixty pavilions and a large church which has become a landmark and is considered one of the major architectural achievements of the Vienna modernistic style. The institution was laid out for 2200 patients and in 1907 the Asylum moved into its new home. The Provincial Council transferred to the Government the former land with all its buildings, as well as some property nearby. Plans were prepared to develop the site with all the medical clinics to be housed in new buildings. The supporter of this project was the well-known surgeon Julius von Hochenegg (1859–1940) whom Wagner-Jauregg called naive in thinking that the Government, in view of the financial circumstances prevailing at the time, would be prepared to build all the clinics straightaway.[36] Other members of the Professorial Board were equally pessimistic.

Wagner-Jauregg felt very strongly that, since the buildings formerly occupied by the Asylum and the First Clinic had been vacated, they should be used, and he proposed that the Clinic at the General Hospital, where conditions were appalling, should be moved there. There was far more accommodation which would allow the Clinic to expand and there were pleasant gardens. Moreover, the move would not take more than a few days. Hochenegg, who had the support of the Director of the General Hospital, opposed Wagner-Jauregg's project. However, it was agreed that an estimate should be obtained for adapting the old buildings so as to render them suitable for the Clinic. This proved to be so high that the responsible authorities hesitated to accept it, and while they procrastinated the project became even more expensive. The Provincial Council was only under an obligation to convey the buildings, but not the installations for lighting and heating, wash rooms and bathrooms, which could have been obtained quite cheaply by the Government. Since it was not prepared to take these over, they were removed, which increased the cost of subsequent adaptation.

Consequently, the Psychiatric Clinic did not at first benefit from the vacation of the old Asylum. However, conditions there worsened to such an extent that they became intolerable: Emil

Kraepelin, who visited the Clinic on the occasion of a Congress for Psychiatric Care in October 1910, describes them in his autobiography as 'shocking'.[37] Patients were penned up in crowded uncomfortable rooms, some in restrain beds placed against the walls (a method for treating agitated patients which Kraepelin found incomprehensible). In a letter dated 5 November 1907 to the Editor of the *Wiener Medizinische Wochenschrift* (the original is in the Library of the City and Province of Vienna – Wiener Stadt- und Landesbibliothek), Adolf Kornfeld (1861–1938),[38] Wagner-Jauregg urged him to draw attention to the urgent need for rebuilding the Clinic. He said he would not mind if he described its conditions as scandalous. Fortunately, a friend of Wagner-Jauregg's, whom he describes as a man with an open mind, von Roretz, became the head of the department responsible for institutions and to him he made his plea that the project for a move to the former asylum be reconsidered. Wagner-Jauregg thought that the original estimate was far too high, and indeed when Roretz asked a young engineer in the building department for a new estimate it turned out to be only about a fifth of the original one and the project was approved.

Thus in 1911 the Second Psychiatric Clinic moved into the far more spacious former Asylum, obtaining wards which had more light and air and also dayrooms and gardens. The difficulty was to find a large enough lecture hall since by that time the subjects of psychiatry and neurology had become obligatory, and a hall that could seat 300 had become necessary. The young engineer responsible for the project had the brilliant idea of converting the chapel of the Asylum into the new lecture hall, leaving the beautiful frescoes which had adorned the chapel untouched.* The rooms which were once the lecture rooms, office and laboratory of the First Clinic became the laboratory which was now in closer proximity to the Clinic it served. From 1911 to the beginning of the First World War in August 1914 the Clinic enjoyed a period of uninterrupted development, which was sadly shattered by the outbreak of hostilities.

---

* Unfortunately, the building no longer exists. It had to make way for the new General Hospital which was developed in the 1970s.

REFERENCES

1 *Zur Geschichte der Psychiatrie in Wien (Psychiatry in Vienna)*. Wien: Brandstätter, 1983.
2 A. Pilcz. Geschichte der klinischen Abteilung (kk.I. Psychiatrische Universitätsklinik) in der Wiener Landes-Irrenanstalt. *Psychiat. Neurol.Wschr.*, 1907, no. 27/28, 231–233.
3 *Wien.Med.Wschr.*, 1874, 24: no. 24, 530–531; no. 25, 558–559.
4 Julius Wagner-Jauregg. Die Wiener psychiatrischen Kliniken. *Wien.Med.Wschr.*, 1936, 86: 481–482.
5 E. Lesky. *Die Wiener Medizinische Schule im 19. Jahrhundert*. Graz-Köln: Hermann Böhlaus, 1965, p. 380.
6 Op.cit. ref 3, p. 558.
7 Ibid. p. 559.
8 Op.cit. ref 2.
9 Richard von Krafft-Ebing. Ueber psychiatrische Kliniken. *Wien. Klin.Wschr.*, 1890, 3: no. 45, 872–875.
10 E. Stransky. *Selbstbiographie*. MS held at Institut für Geschichte der Medizin der Universität Wien.
11 Julius Wagner-Jauregg. *Lebenserinnerungen*. Ed. L. Schönbauer und M. Jantsch. Wien: Springer-Verlag, 1950, p. 56.
12 Ibid. p. 59.
13 J. Starlinger. /Report to the Meeting of the Verein für Psychiatrie und Neurologie on 12 February 1895/ *Wien.Klin.Wschr.*, 1895, 8: no. 31, 565.
14 Op.cit. ref 11, p. 58.
15 Ibid. p. 59; the Obersteiner-Redlich theory was published in *Arb.Inst.Anat.Physiol.Zentralnervensystems Wien Univ.*, 1994, 2: 158–172. Trying to resolve the question who was right the author enlisted the help of Dr Martin Waugh of the General Infirmary at Leeds who in turn approached Professor K. Jellinger, Professor of Neurology and Neuropathology at the Ludwig Boltzmann-Institut für Klinische Neurobiologie in Vienna. It appears that the question who was right, Redlich or Wagner-Jauregg, has not yet been decided.
16 Julius Wagner-Jauregg. Antrittsvorlesung an der psychiatrischen Klinik in der Landesirrenanstalt. *Wien.Klin.Wschr.*, 1893, 6: no. 47, 848–852.
17 Universität Wien. Universitätskalender. Sommersemester 1894.
18 Stransky, op.cit. ref. 10.
19 I.P. Karplus. Eine Plauderei, anlässlich Wagner-Jaureggs 75. Geburtstag. *Wien.Med.Wschr.*, 1932, 82: no. 12, 373–375.

20 F. Hochstetter. Julius Wagner-Jauregg. *Akad.Wiss.Wien.*, *Almanach* für 1941, 91: 197–203.

21 S.L. Last. 'Perspective'. *Psychiat. Bull.*, 1989, 13: 401.

22 O. Pötzl. Julius Wagner von Jauregg. /Obituary/ *Wien.Klin.Wschr.*, 1940, 53: no. 40, 4 p. preceding p. 79.

23 Julius Wagner-Jauregg. Ueber die körperlichen Grundlagen der akuten Psychosen. *Jahrb.Psychiat.*, 1891, 10: 180.

24 Julius Wagner-Jauregg. Ueber Psychosen auf Grundlage gastro-intestinaler Autointoxikation. *Wien.Klin.Wschr.*, 1896, 9: no. 10, 165–170.

25 Wagner-Jauregg, op.cit. ref 11.

26 Paul Roazen. *Helene Deutsch. A Psychoanalyst's Life.* New American Library, 1985.

27 O. Pötzl. Die klinisch-psychiatrischen Anschauungen Wagner-Jaureggs. *Wien.Klin.Wschr.*, 1957, 69. 684–687.

28 Roazen, op.cit. ref 26.

29 Theodor Wagner-Jauregg. *Mein Lebensweg als bioorganischer Chemiker.* Stuttgart: Wissenschaftliche Verlagsgesellschaft, 1985.

30 Stransky, op.cit. ref 10.

31 Last, op.cit. ref 21, p. 402.

32 Wagner-Jauregg, op.cit. ref 11, pp. 62–63.

33 Julius Wagner-Jauregg. Festrede aus Anlass des dreissigjährigen Professorenjubiläums von Hofrat v. Krafft-Ebing. *Wien.Klin.Wschr.*, 1902, 15: no. 12, 318–319.

34 Wagner-Jauregg, op.cit. ref 11, pp. 62–64.

35 Krafft-Ebing, op.cit. ref 9.

36 Wagner-Jauregg, op.cit. ref 11, pp. 65–66.

37 Emil Kraepelin. *Lebenserinnerungen.* Berlin: Springer, 1983, p. 177.

38 Letter from Wagner-Jauregg to Dr Adold Kornfeld, dated 5 November 1907. In the Archives of the Wiener Stadtund Landesbibliothek.

FIVE

THE PROFESSORIAL BOARD

Abrief history of the medical faculty of the University of Vienna was given in the first chapter. As mentioned there, from 1849 the Board of Professors was alone responsible for the direction and administration of teaching, but it was not until 1873 that the Board of Practitioners ceased to be part of the University. That Wagner-Jauregg was anxious to be on the Board that was all powerful in medical education is not surprising. As a full Professor of the University he automatically became a member, and throughout his academic life in Vienna he took an active part in its deliberations and decisions. Not long after his inauguration – indeed only two years after he took office – he was elected Dean of the Medical Faculty, a sign of the high esteem in which he was held by his colleagues.

WAGNER-JAUREGG AS DEAN OF THE MEDICAL FACULTY

For Wagner-Jauregg the appointment as Dean had two distinct advantages: first, responsibility for preparing the proceedings of the Board of Professors and for acting as middleman between it and the Ministry made the Dean an influential figure; secondly, he received a considerable income from fees for examinations and degree awards. At the University of Vienna it had been the custom to elect as Dean theoreticians who relied for their income on their salaries and fees for lectures and examinations. However, when Wagner-Jauregg joined the Board the question was raised whether it was fair to exclude clinicians from the post, and it was decided, as an experiment, to choose a medical practitioner. Thus Wagner-Jauregg was elected, probably because it was thought that, not having a large private practice, he would have time for the work of the Dean; also that he could do with the extra income. However, Wagner-Jauregg was determined to show that it was possible for someone in clinical practice to carry out the duties of Dean without sacrificing too much time to them. It was then the custom for the Dean to be present throughout all examinations, except those in zoology, botany and mineralogy. Often several examinations were taking place at the same time, the practical ones in the morning and the theoretical in the afternoon. Consequently, the Deputy Dean, who was always the former Dean, had to stand in for the Dean. At the end of the semester when there were many examinations two more deputies had to be chosen to act if necessary. These were selected from the non-clinical members of the Board.

When Wagner-Jauregg became Dean he organised matters in such a way that the duties of presiding at examinations were carried out by the Deputy Dean and the two additional deputies. In this way, Wagner-Jauregg had both mornings and afternoons free to devote himself to the affairs of the Dean, his Clinic and even his private practice. Of course, this reduced his income as Dean, because out of it one sixth went to the Deputy Dean and another sixth each to the other two deputies.

Wagner-Jauregg had a very efficient secretary who had had several years' experience in the Dean's office, dating back to the time when Wagner-Jauregg was still a student. Unfortunately, however, it was an open secret that he not only had an open ear for the wishes of students regarding changes in the dates of examinations and the allocation to one or another examiner, but also an open hand. Wagner-Jauregg therefore assumed control of the whole programme of examinations, and students had to apply direct to him – a procedure which involved him in much work. Thus, favouritism came to an end, which was soon appreciated by the better students.

One of the difficulties he encountered concerned the allocation of candidates in subjects in which there was more than one examiner and one was considered stricter than the other. Although he recognised that a candidate who had attended the lectures of one examiner might want to be examined by him, the difficulty was that each examiner had to have the same number of candidates allocated to him. The worst case was in ophthalmology, where nearly all the candidates wanted to be examined by Professor Isidor Schnabel, who was far less strict than Professor Ernst Fuchs. Wagner-Jauregg solved this problem by not publishing the list of candidates to be examined by Schnabel until the same number of candidates had opted for Fuchs. That meant that there was a long waiting list of candidates who wanted to be examined by Schnabel but many who were anxious to take their exams got tired of waiting and were ready to present themselves to Fuchs.

In his *Memoirs* Wagner-Jauregg relates a very unpleasant incident which occurred during his term as Dean on the occasion of the inauguration of the Rector of the University for the academic year 1895–96, the famous lawyer Anton Menger (1841–1906). The student organisations at the time were like cats and dogs. On the one side were the German nationalist fraternities who went in for duelling (after 1870 fraternities practised duelling with swords); on the other were the non-combative catholic unions who refused student duels and did not accept a challenge, though when they were in full dress uniform they too insisted on carrying swords. For some time there had been discussions in the university on whether the non-combative unions should be allowed to wear full dress uniforms at inaugurations, complete with caps, sashes and swords, and whether in that case the duelling fraternities would refuse to attend on such occasions. Finally, it was agreed that the former could do so, and the representatives of the latter promised that they would do nothing to prevent it.

However, at the inauguration when the non-combative catholic unions arrived, they were attacked by students not wearing any distinctive badges, had their caps and sashes ripped off and were prevented from entering the hall. The university attendants and beadles were able to identify some of the miscreants, who were found to be members of the duelling fraternities. Disciplinary proceedings were begun which were to be conducted by the three secular Deans. There was only one medical student among the culprits (medical students did not often join these student corps), and he confessed that he was among the attackers. Wagner-Jauregg reported this to the University Senate, which found him guilty. The student received the *Consilium abeundi*, that is he was threatened with expulsion if found guilty of a misdemeanour again. The deans of the faculties of law and philosophy had to examine several students; the former did not find them guilty (the students got away with lies), and the latter even decided that those attacked were the culprits. The Senate agreed with those verdicts (Wagner-Jauregg calls them comical), and the medical student was the only victim of the affair. However, he did not bear Wagner-Jauregg a grudge.

During Wagner-Jauregg's term as Dean an important matter came before the Board of Professors: the admission of women to medical study. Some professors were in favour, others against. The leading objector was Eduard von Hofmann, Professor of Forensic Medicine, who maintained that if women were given the same opportunities as men, they should also be compelled to do military duty like men and be admitted to the theological faculty. Another opponent of the motion told its leading advocate, the anatomist Emil Zuckerkandl (1849–1910), that he ought to know better than most that women's brains were less developed than those of men.[1] Nevertheless, the majority of the board voted for the admission of women, though Wagner-Jauregg does not say which side he was on. (The medical faculty was not opened to women until 1900).

Another matter to which Wagner-Jauregg gave attention during his term as Dean was further medical education. There had for some time been courses given by medical lecturers for doctors, mostly from abroad, who wished to improve their knowledge, but these were not well organised or publicised. Only during Professor Kundrat's term as Dean was a printed programme issued, announcing two cycles of courses for the holiday months of August and September. When Wagner-Jauregg became Dean he again organised such a course, which required much time and trouble. He continued with this project after he ceased to be Dean, but he arranged for a Committee to be appointed, chosen by the lecturers, to oversee the programme. This was later extended to the whole year, and was continued until the outbreak of the First World War in 1914, to be resumed after the end of the hostilities.

REVISION OF THE MEDICAL SYLLABUS

The revision of the medical syllabus occupied the Professorial Board for some years. Already when he was a member of the Professorial Board at the University of Graz, Wagner-Jauregg had with two other board members sponsored a revision of the syllabus (see pp. 45–46), suggesting the inclusion of paediatrics, psychiatry and dermatology, and reducing the less important subjects such as botany, zoology and mineralogy. The campaign was continued in Vienna and most members of the Faculty with few exceptions voted for the exclusion of zoology and botany. A compromise was reached: a new subject biology was created. Lectures and examinations could be the responsibility of a zoologist or a botanist who would act alternately, and candidates could choose whether they wished to be examined by one or the other. There were also conflicts regarding the inclusion of ancillary subjects such as laryngology, otology and dentistry. Laryngologists, otologists and dentists all wanted their subjects to find a place in the programme of examinations, and in Wagner-Jauregg's opinion they had a better claim than the zoologists and botanists.

Some of the proposals put forward, such as the substitution of biology for botany and zoology and the inclusion of paediatrics as a subject for examination became law in 1899; the specialist subjects of psychiatry and neurology, dermatology, syphilidology and dentistry were included in the syllabus in 1903, as was the separation of histology from anatomy.

REDUCTION OF STUDENT NUMBERS

Not long before the outbreak of the First World War, Wagner-Jauregg was engaged on a project for the reorganisation of medical studies because the number of undergraduates in the medical faculty (not only at the University of Vienna, but at all the Austrian universities) had risen so considerably that the inordinate growth of the medical profession was becoming a problem. Wagner-Jauregg therefore made a suggestion to the Board of Professors which could have been a means for stemming that growth. Most of the professors had been complaining of the scarcity of rooms, of auxiliary staff, of teaching equipment and funds to ensure the proper teaching of the many medical students. During the winter semester of 1913/14 there were 633 medical undergraduates in the first year at the University of Vienna and 1848 at all the seven Austrian universities. Wagner-Jauregg put it to the Board that it was useless to train so many doctors if their number exceeded the need. This was not only a misfortune for them, but also for the patients and society because a lowering of the material standard of doctors would lead to a lowering of moral standards. He therefore proposed that measures should be considered to stop the excessive growth in student numbers. The Board appointed a Committee to consider the whole question with Wagner-Jauregg as referee. As a result it was decided to adopt three measures: first to fix a maximum number of admissions to the medical faculty of the University of Vienna; secondly to refuse admissions to aspirants from a Crownland where a medical faculty existed (thus excluding students from Styria and the Tirol, and also the large influx from Bohemia, Galicia and the Bukovina); and thirdly to raise the fees by a factor of two and a half, in accordance with those charged in Germany. There was some agitation in the press over these proposals. It was claimed that they were intended to reduce the number of Jewish students which at the time amounted to half the total. This was probably the case, for in an unpublished part of the *Memoirs* Wagner-Jauregg refers to the matter as 'trying to settle' the question of the number of Jewish students. There had been violent political demonstrations in 1897 and in 1905 when anti-semitic students rioted in front of the University in an effort to bar Jewish students.

Some members of the Board were not in agreement with these proposals, because for those not doing clinical work lecture and examination fees represented an important source of income. They also objected to the increase in fees because they realised that this would not be granted by the Ministry. However, the Ministry did agree to the maximum number of entrants being fixed at 400 and to the exclusion of those from the Tirol, Styria, Bohemia and Galicia, but not to the increase in fees. None of these decisions were ever acted upon as they were due to come into force in October 1914, and with the outbreak of war in August 1914 the question of an excessive number of medical men no longer arose.

PROBLEMS OF PROMOTION

Problems of promotion and the nomination of candidates for University lectureships caused much excitement and controversy among members of the Board. Proposals for the award of extraordinary professorships also led to much disagreement. Matters of principle were involved: some members believed that too many university lectureships were being created and that there were too many extraordinary professors and those with only the title of Extraordinary Professor. Wagner-Jauregg did not think it was a great misfortune if now and again a university lecturer or extraordinary professor, having been granted either of these titles, ceased to be productive in scientific research.

As the Head of Further Medical Education Wagner-Jauregg was very conscious of the needs of the Faculty. He believed that it was necessary for the Vienna Medical Faculty to attract a great number of teachers in all subjects, because it not only had the task of training doctors of medicine but was also a centre of further medical education. Full Professors usually lacked the time to involve themselves in that important activity and were therefore anxious to avoid holding courses or seminars other than those they were obliged to run.

However, since there were repeated complaints from members of the Board about appointments without any serious proposals for remedying the position, Wagner-Jauregg suggested that the Ministry of Education should be approached with a view to getting its agreement to a change in the rules so that a two-thirds instead of only a simple majority would be required to approve the appointment of a university lecturer and the conferment of the post or the title of Extraordinary Professor. The Board agreed to the proposal, but the Ministry only accepted it in the case of extraordinary professors, rejecting it in the case of university lecturers. It must be remembered that the Ministry had firm control over faculty appointments. Applications for university lectureships occupied the Board of Professors throughout the year. However, proposals for the appointment of extraordinary professors were dealt with only at the end or beginning of the academic year. Since Professors usually proposed their students or assistants, those whose teacher had died or for some other reason had ceased to be a member of the Board were not considered for promotion. Wagner-Jauregg had gained such authority on the Board that he was able to come to the aid of those candidates and propose their names although they did not belong to his specialty. In this way he eventually succeeded in being responsible for the promotion of Julius Donath (1870–1950), who had done much valuable work but whose chief Nothnagel, the Professor of Internal Medicine, had died.

Wagner-Jauregg's *Memoirs* shed some light on the discussions that took place concerning the appointment of university lecturers and promotion to senior posts. His influence on the decisions to confer the *Venia legendi* on some radiologists who became instrumental in furthering that medical specialty, such as Gottwald Schwarz (1880–1959), Guido Holzknecht (1872–1931), Robert Kienböck (1871–1953) and Leopold Freund (1868–1943), was of the utmost importance for the development of radiology. When they first applied, the majority of the members of the Board took the view that radiology was not a subject for which the *Venia legendi* could be granted. The applicants should qualify in a clinical discipline, such as surgery, gynaecology or dermatology, in which they could practise radiology. Wagner-Jauregg, however, realised that to develop radiology effectively it was necessary for practitioners to devote themselves entirely to the subject, which had physical, general biological and technological aspects. He encountered much oppositon among the Professors and in the decisive vote he only had a majority of one. Most Ordinary Professors were against him, but most of the Extraordinary Professors sided with him. Wagner-Jauregg and some of his colleagues eventually succeeded in their proposal for the establishment of a central Institute of Radiology to which all clinics and departments of the General Hospital had access.

In his *Memoirs* Wagner-Jauregg also tells of the intrigues that occurred in connection with appointments to a Chair. It must be remembered that the final decision rested with the Ministry so that, even if the Professors agreed on the choice among themselves, the Minister could still object and appoint whomsoever he chose. Such an incident occurred in 1924 when the Director of the Institute for General and Experimental Pathology died and the Professors proposed an eminent bacteriologist as the first choice for the post. A deputation went to the Ministry, and the short list seemed to have been accepted. However, influenced by an envious member of the Board, the Minister sent a note to the appointing Committee asking whether the experimental aspect of the post had been considered. The answer was in the affirmative, but even another visit to the Ministry failed to bring the hoped-for response. The Minister made several excuses and Wagner-Jauregg, realizing that there was bad will at work, retired from the appointing committee. A provisional solution was found which Wagner-Jauregg considered deplorable. It eventually led to the dissolution of the Institute.

Despite his very active participation in the affairs of the Professorial Board, Wagner-Jauregg turned down the Rectorship of the University of Vienna. It was his turn to be chosen for the academic year 1917–18 because of his seniority, but he had sworn to himself that he would not stand for election by the Academic Senate because of the unpleasant fights that had occurred during elections for the rectorship, and he had often mentioned that he would not accept the position. He kept to the promise he had made to himself and declined to stand, although the philosophers, jurists and theologians would have preferred him to the medical candidate who was eventually chosen.

Wagner-Jauregg was fortunate when it came to the choice of a successor for his Chair and the Directorship of the Clinic. At the University of Vienna it was the rule that a retiring professor could not be a member of the appointing Committee. He could only be asked for advice. Not unnaturally Wagner-Jauregg was most anxious that his successor should continue his work, particularly his malaria therapy. When Friedrich Hartmann (b.1871), Professor at Graz, who was an opponent of the therapy, was proposed, he decided to take all possible steps, both in the Professorial Board and the Ministry, to prevent the appointment. He was successful and his former assistant, Otto Pötzl, who was Professor at the University of Prague, was appointed as his successor.

Further medical education courses

After the war Wagner-Jauregg was asked by the Professorial Board to be reponsible for further medical education courses, particularly those for Americans. In later years the American Medical Association in Vienna flourished and had between 300 and 400 members. This number decreased as a result of the devaluation of the dollar in 1934, and also because of the rapid development of some medical specialties in the United States. Wagner-Jauregg formed a Committee to work out a programme for an international two-week course with three to four lectures in the morning and two to three in the afternoon. The lectures were of one to one and a half hours duration and were to be given be members of the teaching staff who had devoted themselves to a particular subject. The project was greatly furthered by the assistance given by the Editor of the *Wiener Medizinische Wochenschrift*, the Vienna medical weekly, Adolf Kornfeld, who had extensive knowledge of what was happening in the medical field. Those attending the course were invited to an outing to the Semmering, a well-known resort in the hills not far from Vienna, where they were entertained. The success of the project was so great that for a considerable time the courses were held four times a year. After Wagner-Jauregg retired from his Chair in 1928 he could no longer remain Chairman of the Committee and Rudolf Maresch (1868–1936) took over with a Committee chosen by himself. The last course took place in 1937 on the occasion of the celebration of the 150th anniversary of the founding of the Vienna Medical Society.

REFERENCE

[1] Berta Szeps. *My life and history*. London: Cassell, 1936.

SIX

WAGNER-JAUREGG'S FORENSIC ACTIVITIES[1]

One of the tasks of members of the Board of Professors was to give evidence in court, mainly in criminal trials, the criminal courts being legally entitled to demand these reports free of charge. While in Graz Wagner-Jauregg was not often requested to do so, but in Vienna legal advice was asked for by many provinces of the Empire, particularly from Bosnia and Herzegovina. The task of giving evidence in the field of psychiatry was shared by Krafft-Ebing and Wagner-Jauregg. They had repeated disagreements over the question of legal responsibility. From a manuscript which has survived, it is clear that Wagner-Jauregg thought that Krafft-Ebing's opinions were biased and that when evidence was requested of him, he considered it his duty to declare the accused insane and not responsible for his actions; whereas Wagner-Jauregg was not so easily persuaded of the insanity of the accused. In order not to upset a colleague whom he esteemed, to whom he was indebted, and with whom he did not want to come into conflict, he made a point of finding some excuse for not attending meetings of the Committee considering evidence by faculty members when Krafft-Ebing was due to give a report. Thus it came about that accused persons were declared insane when it was Krafft-Ebing's turn to give evidence and usually declared responsible for their actions when it was Wagner-Jauregg's turn. Cases in which mental derangement was obvious were not referred for a report to the Faculty, but were decided by court psychiatrists.

However, an occasion arose, probably shortly before 1902,

when Wagner-Jauregg could no longer avoid a conflict. Both he and Krafft-Ebing had to give an expert opinion. At that time, when Sigmund von Exner (1846–1926) was Dean of the Faculty, the Committee did not include extraordinary professors and lecturers in psychiatry and forensic medicine as was later the case, but only ordinary professors, with Krafft-Ebing and Wagner-Jauregg the only members representing psychiatry. The case on which evidence was requested concerned a Jewish medical student from Bucovina who had been accused of stealing a set of dissecting instruments from a locked locker in the Anatomy Theatre and selling them to an instrument maker. The student had already passed the preliminary examinations of the first Rigorosum. Krafft-Ebing declared him to be insane and therefore not responsible for his actions. This was too much for Wagner-Jauregg and he protested. The other professors were embarrassed, but eventually one suggested that Wagner-Jauregg should examine the accused and report back so that the student had to return to Vienna and submit to Wagner-Jauregg's examination. It soon became clear that he was not insane. When Wagner-Jauregg read to him some of the statements he was purported to have made to Krafft-Ebing, he exclaimed: 'If I had said that, I would be a fool.' Thereupon Wagner-Jauregg invited Krafft-Ebing to examine the student together with him, Krafft-Ebing realised his mistake and, in Wagner-Jauregg's words, 'he behaved like a gentleman'. He took a pencil and without a word crossed out his report and declared himself willing to sign Wagner-Jauregg's. In his account of the incident, Wagner-Jauregg said that Krafft-Ebing accepted the consequences and that this was the reason why he applied for retirement. It is far more likely that the real reason was ill health, since Krafft-Ebing in a letter to a friend in 1894 mentioned that he planned to retire in two years' time.[2] Krafft-Ebing was 62 at the time and according to Wagner-Jauregg looked older, his health having deteriorated owing to too many sleeping drugs. He only survived his retirement for a short time.

As a result, Wagner Jauregg was reponsible for all the reports demanded of the Faculty after Krafft-Ebing's death in 1902. This involved him in much work, particularly as he was extremely conscientious and took great care over them. In the case of psychiatric reports the criminal proceedings had to be studied in detail, and Wagner-Jauregg made use of his right to examine the accused, for which purpose they were brought to his Clinic or to the hospital in the case of prisoners on remand. All these duties made it difficult for him to pursue his scientific work and he therefore applied to the Ministry of Education, with support from the Board of Professors, for a permanent co-referee to be appointed in psychiatric cases. This application was granted and his assistant E. Raimann, who had joined his Clinic in 1899, was chosen for the position, which resulted in his being promoted to the rank of Extraordinary Professor.

When after Krafft-Ebing's death Wagner-Jauregg became responsible for all psychiatric reports, far fewer accused were declared insane and unable to plead, and many court psychiatrists gradually followed his lead. This caused much displeasure to the defending counsels in criminal cases and to the journalists reporting them, as a result of which a popular campaign began in the press against psychiatrists and in particular against Wagner-Jauregg. It resembled the attack levelled against him a few years earlier as a result of a notorious episode in which he got involved in 1896.[3]

THE GIRARDI AFFAIR

The case concerned a famous Austrian comedian, Alexander Girardi (1850–1918), and his wife, a well-known actress with a somewhat doubtful reputation. On 7 December 1896 Wagner-Jauregg was told by a friend, the Professor of Anatomy Emil Zuckerkandl, that he would be called as a consultant to Girardi who had for some time been taking large doses of cocaine and was suspected of being insane. Zuckerkandl, who was a friend of the comedian and his wife, told Wagner-Jauregg that Girardi had become increasingly irritable, particularly towards his wife, whom on one occasion he tried to strangle. Zuckerkandl had witnessed this and when he tackled Girardi about it he explained that he had become very excited because he believed that his wife did not love him. On the evening of 7 December Dr Hoffmann, the physician looking after the staff of the theatre at which Girardi was appearing, called on Wagner-Jauregg and told him that Girardi's irritability was increasing and had become so bad during the past few weeks that he must be considered insane. Girardi treated his wife brutally and created the most frightful scenes before witnesses. On one ocassion, in the presence of Dr Hoffmann, he had pulled out a revolver, shouting to his wife 'We shall not be separated while we are alive.' He was trying to find proof of his wife's unfaithfulness and claimed to have discovered on her writing desk some blotting paper covered with large ink spots, which he was sure represented some secret writing. This made him suspect that his wife had been having affairs with other men. He had also found a tin key in his wife's bedroom which, he thought, provided a clue to the secret writing.

Dr Hoffmann proposed that Wagner-Jauregg come with him on the following day to Girardi's apartment, to which he had access, and be introduced not as a physician (Girardi wanted nothing to do with doctors), but as an expert on secret writings. He expected Girardi to respond readily and reveal his pathological ideas. Dr Hoffmann had no doubt that, if Wagner-Jauregg were to see and speak to Girardi, he would concur with his judgment that he was insane. He told Wagner-Jauregg that he had already booked a room at Svetlin's private asylum and moreover had arranged with the head physician of the Ambulance Corps to be ready on the following day to supervise Girardi's transfer there.

Wagner-Jauregg declared himself ready to examine Girardi the next morning and to decide on his condition and on the measures that ought to be taken, but he insisted that, if a transfer to an asylum were to be considered, he himself could not issue a medical certificate and he would be obliged to insist that a Police Doctor be called in. Girardi's wife, who had for some days been staying at the Hotel Sacher, asked Wagner-Jauregg to call on her as she was anxious to talk to him before he saw her husband. When he visited her she told him about her husband's conduct, especially about his misuse of cocaine, and asked him to accompany her to Svetlin's institution to inspect the room in which her husband was to stay. She was ready to remain with him there, provided the doctors would permit it.

Thus about 10 o'clock on the morning of 8 December Wagner-Jauregg accompanied Dr Hoffmann to Girardi's apartment. When the door was opened a man barred their entry and addressing Dr Hoffmann said that Herr Girardi would not see him. Dr Hoffmann, seeing his plan thwarted, tried to force an entry, but Wagner-Jauregg prevented him from doing so, since they had no right to force their way into somebody else's apartment. At that point Wagner-Jauregg seems to have been in a dither about what to do and acted very unwisely. According to his *Memoirs*, he believed that, on the testimony of the wife, his friend, Professor Zuckerkandl, and Girardi's doctor, Girardi was probably mentally disturbed and very agitated as a result of his marital troubles. He was carrying a weapon which he might use and become a danger to others. Moreover, as a result of his cocaine addiction he might well do himself harm, so Wagner-Jauregg decided that he could not well wash his hands of the affair in case some misfortune occurred and he might justifiably be blamed. He decided therefore to pass the matter over to the authorities who would be entitled to order that Girardi be medically examined and to take any further steps necessary, even against the will of the patient. He went to the Head of the Police and Dr Hoffmann insisted on accompanying him, as he was still anxious to put into effect the arrangements with the Ambulance Corps. They saw the Police President and his Deputy, and after prolonged discussions it was decided, against Wagner-Jauregg's wishes, that the transport that Dr Hoffmann had organised with the Ambulance Corps, and which was still waiting not far from Girardi's apartment, should bring Girardi to the Police Headquarters. In the meantime, Wagner-Jauregg and Dr Hoffmann were asked to write a report on the matter.

In the statement which is reproduced in his *Memoirs* and in a later article, Wagner-Jauregg wrote that he had been led to believe that Herr Girardi had become mentally disturbed, but that he had had no opportunity of examining him.[4] He suggested that he be examined by a Police Doctor. Dr Hoffmann wrote his version on the verso of the same paper, and each signed their own report. The Police Doctor, who had by then been called in, did not think there was any need to add his signature to the statements.

The same afternoon the Police Doctor called on Wagner-Jauregg to tell him that the Ambulance Corps had not found Girardi at home and that he had fled to an unknown destination. The next day the morning papers reported him as missing, but on the following day it was revealed that, accompanied by the man who had barred Wagner-Jauregg's and Dr Hoffmann's entry, he had gone to Katharina Schratt, the famous actress and friend of the emperor Francis Joseph, to ask for her protection. As a result of her intervention, the Police ordered that Girardi be medically examined, whereupon both the Police Doctor and the chief forensic psychiatrist found that Girardi was not mentally disturbed and was free to go where he liked.

Now all hell was let loose in the press and an attack was mounted against psychiatrists. It was claimed that patients in asylums, particularly in private asylums, were detained through the machinations of their enemies with the aid of psychiatrists, and that Wagner-Jauregg, without examining Girardi, had given testimony to confine him to an asylum in order to please his wife. The newspapers printed Wagner-Jauregg's version of the affair, but continued to adhere to theirs on the following day. A well-known journalist and writer, Felix Salten, demanded Wagner-Jauregg's dismissal from his post, and a most abusive article appeared in one of the papers.[5]

Girardi sued Dr Hoffmann for attempted deprivation of freedom, and Wagner-Jauregg was called as a witness. The matter never came to court because of a lack of evidence, but Wagner-Jauregg gained the impression that the examining judge had come to the conclusion that Girardi's behaviour had justified the suspicion of mental disturbance. The well-known Professor of Nervous Diseases, Moriz Benedikt (1835–1920), in an article in a legal journal, discussed the affair without naming Girardi.[6] He thought that, as a clever comedian, Girardi had acted the frenzied and hallucinating madman to get himself out of an awkward situation. When his doctor took him seriously and the comedy threatened to become a tragedy by his internment in an asylum, he gave up his act and claimed to be the victim of an intrigue.

The case of the bank note forger

Wagner-Jauregg's standing with the press improved somewhat after his part in a case in which he caused the defence serious embarrassment in criminal proceedings in open court. It concerned a forger of bank notes who, with several accomplices, was on remand. The accused simulated insanity but the psychiatrists believed that he was not insane, and consequently the case had to be proceeded with. However, at each hearing the accused was taken ill, almost fainted and the court doctor present declared him unfit to plead. The proceedings had to be adjourned, which was an embarrassment as the case was being tried by a jury and the President of the Court was in despair. He called for a psychiatrist, a former assistant of Wagner-Jauregg's, Dr Elzholz, who became convinced that the fainting fit was not simulated because the accused showed greatly enlarged pupils. This increased the discomfort of the President who asked that Wagner-Jauregg, as the author of the specialist report, be invited to attend the next sitting and with some reservations Wagner-Jauregg agreed. He noticed that during the proceedings the accused repeatedly put his handkerchief to his nose without blowing it, once again becoming ill. Wagner-Jauregg noted the enlarged pupils and for him the case was clear: it was cocaine that caused the accused to feel ill, but he had to prove this to the jury. He needed a *corpus delicti* and he therefore asked that the accused be taken to a room where he could be examined. Meanwhile, the sitting had to be adjourned, whereupon not only the warder, but also the defence lawyer, whom Wagner-Jauregg did not trust, and a whole 'pack' of journalists followed the accused and Wagner-Jauregg into the private room. All the time Wagner-Jauregg, while examining the accused, kept his eyes on the jacket which the latter had removed and on the pocket in which the handkerchief had been put. Rather abruptly he shouted at the President of the Court to have all the people who had no business to be in the room removed. In the resulting commotion he reached out to the jacket of the accused and pulled out the handkerchief.

Wagner-Jauregg returned to the Court and opened the handkerchief before the jury: it contained dried up powder which he suspected to be cocaine, as the accused had shown all the symptoms of cocaine poisoning. His suspicion was confirmed when the powder was analysed and found to be cocaine. As a result the accused was sent to prison for eight years.

The murder of the Prime Minister

In his recollections Wagner-Jauregg recounts a famous case in which he had to give expert evidence that caused him more work than any other in his career. It concerned the murder on 21 October 1916 of Count Stürgk, the Austrian Prime Minister, who was shot in the dining-room of one of the best hotels in Vienna by Dr Friedrich Adler (b. 1879). He was the son of the well-known and respected leader of the Social Democrats and founder of the daily paper *Arbeiter Zeitung (Workers' Daily)*, Victor Adler (1852–1918). From his youth Friedrich Adler had been brought up on the ideals of the socialist movement. At the time of the outbreak of the First World War he was secretary of the Party, and he had expected its leaders to oppose the war, even at the risk of sacrificing their lives. Instead, most party members and the population as a whole showed their patriotism and stood by the Emperor and the Government. Friedrich Adler came into increasing opposition with the leaders of the Party, including his father, and began to plan an attack against someone in power. He wanted to become a martyr for the cause and thus help the rejuvenation of the socialist movement. He first thought of the Minister of Justice, then the State Attorney, and finally Count Stürgk, the Prime Minister. Two events strengthened his resolution: the first was a decree, issued by Count Stürgk on the day before the murder, forbidding assemblies demanding the recall of Parliament. (Count Stürgk had dissolved Parliament in 1914.) The second was a telephone conversation with a member of the Vienna Philosophical Faculty who was in sympathy with socialist policy, during which he learned that Count Stürgk regularly lunched in the dining-room of the Hotel Meissl and Schaden, one of the best hotels in Vienna.

Friedrich's father, Victor Adler, and the defending lawyers tried to prove that he was insane, maintaining that he had suffered from time to time from mental disturbances and that there was a history of mental illness on both his father's and his mother's side. In view of the importance of the case, it was referred to the psychiatric faculty without a previous examination by the court psychiatrists, as was usual, and Wagner-Jauregg was called on for an expert opinion. In his recollections Wagner-Jauregg gives a detailed account of the mental histories of several of the Adler family. However, he firmly believed that in forensic cases mental derangement of the accused could not be proved by heredity, but only by personal examination and observation. Consequently, he had to concern himself with the state of mind of Friedrich Adler, whom no one had ever considered to be insane. Instead, he suffered from what we call psychosomatic symptoms which were then diagnosed as chronic myocarditis. Wagner-Jauregg, however, greatly doubted this diagnosis, as Friedrich Adler was able to undertake strenuous mountain climbs when his states of depression ceased. Moreover, the latter were never sufficiently serious to affect his scientific and political activities. According to Wagner-Jauregg, his deed was not due to emotional disturbance but to political conviction.

Here Wagner-Jauregg's recollections end, but it is clear that he did not declare the accused insane since Friedrich Adler was convicted of the murder of Count Stürgk at his trial in May 1917 and sentenced to death. He delivered a rousing speech and an extraordinary indictment of prevailing government methods, to the effect that the death sentence was commuted to life imprisonment. He was freed by an amnesty early in November 1918, shortly before Austria became a Republic.

THE REFORM OF INSANITY REGULATIONS

In Austria the first attempts to create a generally acceptable law on insanity were made under Maria Theresa, and in 1812 a general code for Austria was put into effect. The paragraph which dealt with interdiction stated that only those should be considered insane or imbecile who had been judged so by court-appointed medical experts and whose behaviour had been carefully observed. The regulation that the Court had to appoint the medical experts was made in order to exclude medical men who lacked knowledge or who had been bribed.

Although the civil law provided protection against unjustified interdiction, the admission to an asylum remained a matter for the administration. The efforts made during the years 1859–74 to create a lunacy law were largely due to the Director of the Asylum of Lower Austria, Ludwig Schlager and also to J. von Mundy (1822–94) and H.H. Beer (1798–1873), Professor of Forensic Medicine. They are described in some detail in a work on the reform of the legislation and the proposals for a projected new law by S. Türkel, published in 1907.[7] Two orders issued in 1874 and 1878 by the Ministry of the Interior in agreement with the Ministry of Justice had not dealt with the field of lunacy legislation in an exhaustive manner and had left many loopholes.

According to the order of 1874, the admission of a patient to an asylum had to be notified to a Court of first instance within twenty-four hours. Although this provided protection against wrongful internment in an asylum, there was much mistrust of psychiatrists, who were thought to be ready to accept sane persons in asylums, either to deprive them of their rights with criminal intention, or to save them from the criminal law. The publicity following the Girardi episode added to the clamour in the press for a revision of such insanity regulations as then existed. After Wagner-Jauregg took over the direction of the First Psychiatric Clinic of Vienna in 1893, a member of parliament proposed in every session the creation of a lunacy law, and much attention was paid to the question by the daily press. Eventually, the authorities were led to consider the introduction of a law that would ensure the protection of both the mentally ill and the general public. As a result, the Ministry of the Interior and the Ministry of Justice decided in 1898 to ask the Senior Health Council, which acted as adviser to the Government, for a report on the reform of the lunacy legislation, and Wagner-Jauregg was asked to act as a referee. He believed that, in view of the importance of the freedom of the person, lunacy matters should be regulated by legislation rather than ministerial orders. The two principal objects of such a law should be: (1) the protection of the personal rights of the insane person, and (2) the right of the insane to proper care and treatment; the first object concerned the legal authorities, the second would involve administrative action. Some of the difficulties seem to have arisen from the fact that asylums were the responsibility of the provincial governments, so that the legal protection of the insane was subject to the law of the province concerned rather than to that of the State. In his report, of which an account is given in Türkel's book, Wagner-Jauregg examined the ways in which the law, as it operated at the time, was insufficient to protect the insane. As far as legal protection was concerned, it was based solely on the civil law, which made insufficient provision regarding the rights and duties of guardians and ignored the care of the person. A duty to notify admission to an asylum should be included in the statutes, as well as the conditions for admission to and discharge from asylums. The care of patients in private institutions needed to be regulated as well, as should the relation of the insane with the criminal law. Finally, Wagner-Jauregg proposed that the Senior Health Council should recommend that the Ministry of the Interior, in agreement with the Ministry of Justice, should entrust a Commission of Enquiry, consisting of representatives of the two Ministries and the Senior Health Council, with the preliminary work for the drafting of a lunacy law. This recommendation was accepted by the Senior Health Council on 8 July 1899.

A few months prior to that decision, in January 1899, Wagner-Jauregg had been appointed to serve permanently on the Council. At the time there was no psychiatrist on that body and it had been expected that Krafft-Ebing, the director of the Second Psychiatric Clinic, the most senior psychiatrist in the country and author of a textbook on forensic psychiatry, would be appointed to that position. However, according to Wagner-Jauregg, Krafft-Ebing had enemies both in government circles and among the Board of Professors, and so Wagner-Jauregg was appointed instead. He believed that he owed the appointment to friends on the Council and among the Professors, notably Eduard von Hofmann who had been much impressed by the report on alcoholism which Wagner-Jauregg had written for Leidesdorf when the latter was unable to produce it because of illness.

The Commission of Enquiry appointed by the Senior Health Council included the leading psychiatrists not only of Vienna, but also from other parts of the Empire. Among them were Wagner-Jauregg and Krafft-Ebing. The work by Türkel mentioned earlier gives a detailed account of the proceedings of the Commission during

1901 and 1902. It is clear from this that Wagner-Jauregg was the leading light in the discussions, being the most prominent speaker at every session and expressing his views at greater length than the other members of the Commission. His opinions seem to have found acceptance, notably his suggestion that the questions to be discussed be considered under nine main headings: (1) the duty of notification; (2) the supervision of the care of the insane; (3) the creation of state asylums; (4) private asylums; (5) admission to an asylum; (6) the transfer of the insane; (7) discharge and leave from asylums; (8) interdiction and guardianship; and (9) care of insane criminals and the criminally insane. A referee should be appointed to report on each of these groups, with Wagner-Jauregg to be the referee for the question of admission to asylums and the protection against unjustified internment, and, together with Professor Moriz Benedikt, on the treatment of the criminally insane. Krafft-Ebing was to report on the interdiction of the insane; his suggestion that representatives of private asylums should be invited to join the Commission, was opposed, particularly by Wagner-Jauregg.

The shortened version of Wagner-Jauregg's report on the first question occupies seven closely-printed pages and that on the second four pages. In the first, Wagner-Jauregg urged that application for admission should be facilitated and not delayed. It could be granted without the intervention of the authorities to close relatives living in the same household. Insanity must be confirmed by a medical certificate, issued not earlier than fourteen days before admission, though in obvious and urgent cases the insane person could be admitted without a certificate, and voluntary entry into an institution should be made possible. To avoid sane persons being admitted, the director of the institution concerned should be obliged to notify every admission to the law office within twenty-four hours, except in the case of a voluntary admission. However, there should be a duty to notify if the voluntary stay in the asylum became a forced one. Psychiatrists should be subject to control by the legal authorities to prevent misuse of their powers. Every adult insane person admitted to an asylum must be examined by two experts who had had at least four years' experience in a psychiatric clinic or similar institution, and who should not be on the staff of the asylum in question. These measures should prevent wrongful admissions to asylums and unjustified detention could be avoided if any request by the patient for re-examination of his mental state was granted.

The joint report with Professor Benedikt[8] on the treatment of the criminally insane, reproduced in Türkel's book, urged the provision of special institutions for them, arguing against annexes to prisons or asylums. Two categories of persons who should be sent to these special institutions were: (1) individuals involved in criminal proceedings who were found to be insane; and (2) individuals convicted of a crime who became insane while detained. However, there were some among these two categories who might be admitted to an ordinary asylum without risk, because they would not disturb the order of that institution nor exert unfavourable influence on the other patients. On the other hand, asylums must be freed of patients with criminal tendencies. Admission to an institution for the criminally insane would have to be not only on the strength of medical evidence but also by decision of the legal authorities.

Whereas asylums were under the control of the provinces, the institutions for the criminally insane should be under that of the State. A different discipline would be necessary for them and the provinces should be obliged to defray the cost of maintenance for those in the State institutions, otherwise it was feared that there might be a conflict of competence between the two official bodies.

The meetings of the Commission took place during the years 1901 and 1902. Already in 1901 Wagner-Jauregg had written a series of five articles,[9] published in one of the Vienna medical weeklies, in which he dealt at some length with the reform of the insanity legislation. His immediate purpose was to oppose the campaign initiated in the Vienna daily press urging the reform of the lunacy laws and demanding that certification of the mentally ill and their admission into asylums should in future not depend on medical, but on lay evidence, that is on the decision of a Commission of independent men who enjoyed the confidence of their fellow citizens. The campaign was supported by some well-known personalities and in the articles mentioned above Wagner-Jauregg severely attacked the initiator of the campaign, which he called 'the baiting of psychiatrists'. This was a certain Eduard August Schroeder who had previously published two books on the reform of the lunacy system, inspired, according to Wagner-Jauregg, by a passionate dislike of the psychiatric profession. Schroeder imputed sinister motives to the opinions and actions of psychiatrists who, in his view, were biased and who would like to declare everyone to be mentally disturbed. He claimed that innumerable victims of the lunacy law, as it then existed, had been unjustifiably held in asylums and had committed suicide rather than live under the dreadful curse of an invented mental illness. Thousands would have died a natural death if they had not been deprived of their freedom.

Schroeder called psychiatry a pseudo-science and accused psychiatrists of making every effort to retain and widen their power, often rendering their patients insane through their treatment. Wagner-Jauregg believed that Schroeder found the existence of mental illness uncomfortable and wanted to show that its apparently frequent occurrence was due to the prejudiced opinion of psychiatrists. In Schroeder's opinion, the only justifiable aim of psychiatry was to provide proof of insanity through somatic examination. As Wagner-Jauregg commented, how such an examination could prove that a person was sane and how anyone could judge that a person was insane purely by somatic examination was beyond his understanding.

Wagner-Jauregg believed that the agitation against psychiatrists was due to the publicity given to a few cases in which sane persons had been sent to an asylum because their behaviour had led inexperienced physicians to believe that they were insane. (It was then still not obligatory for medical students to attend a course in psychiatry.) However, most of the cases in which unjustified internment in an asylum was claimed concerned those whose criminality had made it necessary for them to be deprived of their freedom.

The source of all the difficulties seemed to be the problem of determining the border-line between insanity and criminality. Wagner-Jauregg considered it a mistake to send a criminal to an asylum because of his pathological nature. In any case, he thought that these problems were better kept from lay men, since experts in both medicine and law had tried in vain to find a satisfactory solution to them. He argued forcibly and vehemently against the competence of a lay jury to decide on whether a person ought to be certified.

In the third of his articles Wagner-Jauregg dealt with the legal protection of the insane, which he considered one of the most important objects of insanity legislation, and he outlined the views contained in his report to the Commission for the revision of the lunacy law described earlier. They related to the admission to asylums and the criteria governing the restriction of personal freedom. He also discussed the protection of the patient's property. His fourth article was devoted to problems associated with the criminally insane as set out in the joint report, with Benedikt, to the Commission. In it Wagner-Jauregg again stressed the need for the establishment of institutions for the criminally insane, and discussed the question whether they should be independent or annexed to asylums or prisons and which individuals ought to be cared for in these. In this connection, he quoted the proposals contained in the draft for the French insanity legislation, which he thought might be applicable to the Austrian situation. According to these, the State should establish several institutions for the criminally insane. To these should be sent: (1) those accused who had been acquitted because of unsound mind; (2) those sentenced who became insane while in prison; and (3) insane persons who while in the asylum committed a crime against the person. Wagner-Jauregg did not believe that all persons mentioned under (1) and (2) should necessarily be sent to these institutions and that these provisions should not be obligatory but facultative. The main aim was to include those who, apart from the mental disturbance, showed criminal tendencies and/or had a criminal past.

In the final article of the series Wagner-Jauregg dealt with alcoholism in relation to the insane, with particular reference to the proceedings of the International Congress on Alcoholism in 1901. One of the questions discussed concerned the way in which the asylum, through detention and forced abstinence, could contribute to the cure of an alcoholic. Wagner-Jauregg deplored the attack of Professor August Forel (1848–1931), a former Director of Burghölzli (the well-known Swiss asylum), whom he called the apostle of abstinence, against the Director of the Vienna Asylum, Dr Tilkovsky, for having discharged alcoholics too soon. In Wagner-Jauregg's view the task of the asylum could only be the cure and treatment of mental diseases caused by alcoholism, not the cure of alcohol addiction itself. Support for this view was the movement for the creation of sanatoria for the cure of drinkers which would not be necessary if the asylum could cure alcohol addiction.

In his lecture to the Congress[10] Wagner-Jauregg dealt with the toxicology of alcohol and symptoms of abstinence after chronic misuse of alcohol, particularly the delirium alcoholicum which he regarded as a consequence of the sudden withdrawal of alcohol. He encountered a storm of protest from fanatic teetotallers and sanatoria where abstinence was practised.

According to Wagner-Jauregg's reminiscences, the reports submitted to the Commission of Enquiry during 1901/2 were discussed in a plenary session of the Senior Health Council and the complete minutes were submitted to the Ministry of the Interior, which in turn passed them on to the Ministry of Justice and also to

Parliament. It transpired that there was no government intention to create a comprehensive lunacy law at the time, only to introduce a law for the protection of the insane against unjustified internment. The question of the criminally insane would be dealt with in conjunction with the planned reform of the criminal law.

The Minister of Justice at the time was much concerned with the proposal for a law for the protection of the insane in conjunction with a law for the application and cancellation of interdiction. Wagner-Jauregg felt that his attitude did not differ greatly from that of Schröder whom Wagner-Jauregg had attacked in the articles mentioned above. It is clear that some people wanted lay men involved in the process, whereas psychiatrists were insistent that only the view of medical experts should prevail. When the law was eventually drafted it was submitted to the Director of the Office of Public Health and to Wagner-Jauregg as the representative of the Senior Health Council. They had many conferences with the civil servant in charge of the relevant department of the Ministry. They both found the draft unacceptable not only because its provisions would delay and make more complicated the admission of a person to the asylum, but also because it envisaged the appointment of a 'trusted person', not necessarily a medical man or a lawyer, who had to be invited to all proceedings and allowed to consult and copy all documents.

The draft did, however, contain some welcome suggestions, probably largely due to the work of the Commission of 1901/2 and Wagner-Jauregg's reports. One of these provided for the grant of voluntary entry into asylums, which would do away with the need to notify the legal authorities of all admissions. This would also make it possible for insane persons to be admitted to other institutions – for example, to sanatoria and hydropathic establishments, which had previously not been allowed to admit the insane. They had therefore, to circumvent this restriction, described them in their records as suffering from some physical illness.

When the legislative proposals became known Wagner-Jauregg, through the Society for Psychiatry in Vienna, gave asylum and forensic psychiatrists, as well as those interested in legal reform, the opportunity to discuss them. The Society organised regular meetings, mostly in Vienna, to which Austrian psychiatrists were invited and where questions about the regulation of mental health matters could be discussed. In the manuscript in which he relates these activities, Wagner-Jauregg stresses that questions relating to the organisation of the system dealing with the insane had to be considered from three standpoints: that of the psychiatrist, that of the legislator and that of the lay man whose relatives might become psychiatric patients. It was necessary to bear in mind the limits on what could be achieved, but most psychiatrists lacked any ability to see things from more than one standpoint. Indeed, they considered as an insult the suggestion that their admission of an insane person needed to be checked.

Wagner-Jauregg's important and influential thinking on the question of responsibility is contained in his report to the Austrian Meeting of Psychiatrists in October 1907,[11] in which he made a number of suggestions regarding the formulation of the new law. In his opinion, it should state that the medical expert could only pronounce on the mental derangement, but that it was a matter for the judge to decide the question of responsibility; similarly, only the judge could decide on the question of free-will if that were to be introduced into the law. He thought that only a pronounced degree of mental derangement should lead to the insanity defence, and that responsibility should not be judged in general, but in respect of the gravity and nature of the punishable offence. In cases of drunkenness, the expression 'complete intoxication' should be avoided, and responsibility be judged in respect of the punishable offence. Wagner-Jauregg proposed that the concept of 'diminished responsibility' should be included in the new law, and he urged again that special provision should be made for the treatment of criminally insane persons.

For the paragraph dealing with the insanity defence Wagner-Jauregg proposed the following wording: 'The person who at the time of the crime is unable to realise the wrongness of the deed because of mental derangement, deaf-muteness or drunkenness, or because he had no free-will, should not be punishable. It is the task of the judge, not of the expert witness, to determine this. The absolution from punishment should not apply if the accused knows from experience that he might perform misdeeds when totally drunk.'[12]

In an article on pathological compulsive actions, written a few years later,[13] Wagner-Jauregg examined criminal actions arising from pathological causes – such as sexual urges, sadism, or arson – which, in his view, were the product of pathological brain activity. It was sometimes difficult, for example, to draw the line between thieves and kleptomaniacs. However, he concluded that proof of compulsion was not sufficient to absolve the culprit from responsibility.

Wagner-Jauregg was very hurt when in 1910 two of his former assistants, J. Schweighofer and J. Starlinger, probably aggrieved because they had not been included in the discussions with the Ministries, founded a new society composed of asylum psychiatrists from the whole Empire, in opposition to the Society for Psychiatry in Vienna, to discuss questions of insanity regulations at places outside Vienna. Wagner-Jauregg felt as if he had been attacked from behind and withdrew more and more from discussions other than those with criminal aspects, but he was still frequently consulted by the Ministries. For example, as late as 1926, in a report requested and approved by the Senior Health Council, he urged once again the need to establish institutions for the criminally insane, particularly as the number of those found insane was expected to increase if the concept of diminished responsibility was introduced into the criminal law.

At last, in 1916, a law on interdiction was passed as an Imperial Order. It provided for two kinds of interdiction, a complete and a limited one; for notification to the courts of admissions, other than voluntary, with obligatory examination of the insane person by a judge and two experts; and for permission to admit insane persons to nursing homes and sanatoria. The 'trusted person' of the earlier draft, to which Wagner-Jauregg had objected, had disappeared and been replace by a 'representative', presumably a lawyer.

When, in 1937, the Honorary Doctorate of Law was awarded to Wagner-Jauregg, the Dean of the Faculty praised his activities as expert witness in criminal cases and referred to his reports as masterpieces of forensic psychiatry. Above all, he stressed that his work laid the foundation for the 1912 draft of the Austrian criminal law.[14] In an appreciation of Wagner-Jauregg on the occasion of the 100th anniversary of his birth, H. Hoff (1897–1969) gave a full account of his work in forensic psychiatry, a field in which his name had been largely forgotten because all his ideas had become integrated into Austrian law and were now regarded as self-evident.[15]

REFERENCES

[1] This chapter is largely based on two manuscripts containing reminiscences, found among Wagner-Jauregg's papers, entitled 'Psychiatrisch forensische Tätigkeit' and 'Forensische Psychiatrie

   – Irrengesetzgebung'. They are not dated but internal evidence suggests that they were written after Wagner-Jauregg's retirement, probably in the 1930s. They are kept at Institut für Geschichte der Medizin der Universität Wien.

[2] Renate Hauser. Richard von Krafft-Ebing. Thesis, University of London, 1992.

[3] An account by Wagner-Jauregg of the Girardi affair is in his *Lebenserinnerungen* (Wien: Springer Verlag, 1950), pp. 107–113, and in *Psychiat.Neurol.Wschr.*, 1933, 12: 145–147.

[4] Ibid.

[5] Felix Salten. *Neue Freie Presse*, December 1896.

[6] Moriz Benedikt. *Allgemeine österreichische Gerichtszeitung*, 1901.

[7] Siegfried Türkel. *Die Reform des Oesterreichischen Irrenrechtes*. Leipzig und Wien: Franz Deuticke, 1907.

[8] Türkel, op.cit. ref 7, pp. 134–138.

[9] Julius Wagner-Jauregg. Zur Reform des Irrenwesens. *Wien.Klin.Wschr.*, 1901, 14: no. 12, 293–296; no. 13, 324–326; no. 21, 518–521; no. 30, 720–723.

[10] Ibid. 720–723.

[11] Oesterreichischer Irrenaerztetag. *Jahrb.Psychiat.Neurol.*, 1909, 29: 390–399.

[12] Julius Wagner-Jauregg. Der Unzurechnungsfähigkeitsparagraph im ÖStGE. *Österr.Zentralbl.juridische Praxis*, 1907, 25: no. 11/12.

[13] Julius Wagner-Jauregg. Krankhafte Triebhandlungen. *Wien.Klin.Wschr.*, 1912, 25: no. 11, 403–408.

[14] Ferdinand Kadecka. Verleihung des Ehrendoktorates der Rechte an Herrn Universitätsprofessor Dr Julius von Wagner-Jauregg. *Wien.Klin.Wschr.*, 1937, 50: no. 20, 657–658.

[15] H. Hoff. Zum Geburtstag Wagner-Jauregs. *Wien.Z.Nervenheilk.*, 1958, 14: no. 1, 8–10; also *Wien.Med.Wschr.*, 1957, 107: no. 29/30, 618–621.

SEVEN

THE WAR AND ITS AFTERMATH: FREUD AND WAGNER-JAUREGG

When war broke out in August 1914 Wagner-Jauregg happened to be on holiday in Carinthia. He had to return to Vienna immediately – fortunately on the first day after the declaration of war the trains were still running as usual – because he was the head of the academic riding school and was responsible for eighteen horses allocated to the school by the Government which had to be returned forthwith. At the time, Wagner-Jauregg was over 57 years old and had no military responsibilities, having left the reserve in 1892 after serving the obligatory period of service.

Since many doctors were called up, the clinic became short of staff. In a letter to an anonymous colleague which was among some medical letters auctioned at Sothebys in 1988, Wagner-Jauregg said how greatly the staff had been reduced, mentioning Dr Pötzl, Frau Dr Freund, Dr Fahrmann and a Russian doctor as those remaining. To carry on the work of the Clinic Wagner-Jauregg was allowed to designate as indispensable one assistant who would not have to join the forces. At the time the father of Dr Pötzl, his first assistant, was so seriously ill that it would have been hard on him to leave and Wagner-Jauregg therefore declared him to be indispensable. Pötzl assisted his chief in the running of the clinic for men, whereas in that for women he was helped by a woman doctor. In his *Memoirs* Wagner-Jauregg did not mention the name of the woman doctor and it is not clear whether this was the Frau Dr Freund mentioned in the letter referred to above, or Helene Deutsch, who – according to Paul Roazen[1] – was preparing to join the staff of the Clinic, probably in about 1913. She was supposed to serve on the women's and children's wards and rose to the position as Wagner-Jauregg's assistant in charge of the women's division. It is strange that Wagner-Jauregg did not mention her by name as they seemed to be on very good terms: Helene liked him and spoke very highly of him. In 1919 when a friend of hers, Paul Schilder (1886–1940), had come back from the war, she left the Clinic for his sake, thinking that Wagner-Jauregg would prefer him to her, and also because she had become a disciple of Freud. It may well have been for that reason that Wagner-Jauregg preferred to forget her, although Schilder too was a disciple of Freud and – according to his biographer[2] – was considered his favourite. Unhappily, Wagner-Jauregg and Schilder were two strong, but dissimilar, personalities and friendship between them ceased. Nevertheless, Schilder received the title of Professor in 1925 on the recommendation of Wagner-Jauregg, the first time that anybody connected with psychoanalysis was promoted at the University of Vienna. Also, according to Dr Last[3], Wagner-Jauregg allowed Schilder to lecture on psychoanalysis, the only German-speaking Clinic where a psychoanalyst was permitted to do so.

Alfred Fuchs (1870–1927) was the assistant in charge of the Neurology Clinic, which was for men only. It had to be increased continually during the war so that eventually it contained 900 beds, mainly occupied by those who had suffered head injuries. In addition to his work at the Clinics, Wagner-Jauregg had many other responsibilities. At one of the army hospitals, a university lecturer in internal medicine had been put in charge of the neurology department. As the field was new to him, he asked Wagner-Jauregg to assist him in writing reports on the injured and Wagner-Jauregg at first went to the hospital every day and later two or three times a week. Moreover, he had to give his expert advice on injured and sick soldiers and was concerned with the two institutions of the Rothschild Foundations which had been requisitioned as army hospitals. Although the medical direction of one was in the hands of Friedrich Sölder (1867–1943) and the other of Professor Redlich, his former assistant, Wagner-Jauregg was Vice-President of the Council of the Foundation; and since its President, Alfons Rothschild, had joined the forces, he was responsible for the administration of both. His private practice also took up much of his time, although there were few paying patients. Since he had decided, as a kind of voluntary war service, to treat free of charge all military personnel – from privates to field marshall, regardless of their nationality – he could not complain of a lack of patients!

The Neurology Clinic at the General Hospital became increasingly busy. Among the first cases were patients who had lost their speech as a result of shell-shock, although they understood what was said to them and could communicate in writing. Wagner-Jauregg believed[4] that mutism as a result of shell-shock, sometimes accompanied by deafness, might not be entirely psychological but caused by physical lesions, due to mechanical damage to hearing. Often when speech returned it was accompanied by stuttering. Mutism was generally affected by psychological influences. Cases of speech loss were cured quickly even among those who had spent weeks and months in other hospitals without improvement. The therapies used were psychological and in some cases they were somewhat intimidating, involving isolation, bland but sufficient diet, unpleasant medication or electrotherapy (Faradism applied with a brush). The question was raised whether the trauma of shell-shock was due to a psychologically caused disturbance of nerve function or a physical effect. Wagner-Jauregg did not adopt the view that the physical effects of shell-shock could be discounted. On the other hand, the quick recovery from the disturbances showed that therapeutic measures, which might be described as psychological, also caused the somatic components of the shock to disappear.

Cases of speech loss as a result of shell-shock gradually disappeared from the Clinic, because they were dealt with at hospitals nearer the front. On the other hand, the number of disorders of movement of the lower extremities, mostly associated with trembling, increased rapidly. Wagner-Jauregg was able to distinguish between the genuinely sick and those that simulated illness. He recognised the psychogenic causes and the nature of shell-shock and was aware of the hysterical and hysteroid nature of *Myotonoklonia trepidans*, the trembling of legs, in which, as he said, 'the shell generally only exploded in the anamnesis', and which represented a flight mechanism into sickness. He realised that there were cases that required individual psychotherapy and that often there was no noticeable dividing line between 'those who want to but cannot and those who can but do not want to'. He knew that often unethical and asocial components were part of hysterical mechanisms, and that in these cases a therapy of energetic discipline was indicated, not psychoanalytic treatment.

At the Clinic there were countless cases of psychologically caused paralytic and spastic disturbances of movement, ranging from complete paralysis with or without rigidity to more or less severe trembling of limbs. The trembling of legs became a nervous epidemic, relieving its sufferers from the obligation to do war service. These patients were treated in the same way as those who had lost their speech, mainly with electrotherapy. Their recovery was slower and consequently stronger Faradic currents, applied by brush to the sides of the toes, had to be used. In his *Memoirs* Wagner-Jauregg describes how when he himself performed the therapy he always applied the current to his hand first, so as to show the patient that the pain caused by the treatment could easily be withstood. He recommended this method to the other physicians in the Clinic who had to carry out the treatment, but not one of them made use 'of my recommendation'.[5]

The type of electrotherapy in question did not originate at the time of the First World War, but had been extensively used during the second half of the nineteenth century. A number of books were published on the subject during the 1850s and 1860s, and around the turn of the century there were three hospitals in Vienna where this treatment was being carried out. It is quite different from the electric shock treatment which is used nowadays and it is no longer practised. The medical apparatus consisted of one or more galvanic elements which served as sources of electricity and provided an induced current. The alternating Faradic current produced in this apparatus was not in any way dangerous to the healthy body. A secondary apparatus was used when the source of electricity was power from the public network, of 110–120 volts, because this voltage had to be reduced for medical purposes. Current from a differential electrode was used for therapeutic purposes, usually taking the form of brush-like electrodes. This type of secondary apparatus was not used at Wagner-Jauregg's Clinic because of the danger of accidents.

With this method, patients suffering from trembling were cured very quickly – so much so, that the military authorities sent more and more patients afflicted with this disorder to the Clinic. This was unwelcome to Wagner-Jauregg, because many of the patients were neither pleased nor grateful, since they would have preferred to remain unfit until the end of the war to escape further military service. Agitation against the method began to mount. To understand this popular unrest, which became increasingly vociferous at the end of the war, it must be remembered that the break-up of the Empire had brought about a complete upheaval in the life of what remained of Austria itself, causing a search for scapegoats which was seized upon by the Socialist press. On 11 December 1918 there appeared in the Social-Democratic weekly *The Free Soldier* an article under the title 'The electric torture', in which the medical profession was accused of supporting militarism and cruelty against soldiers during the war. In particular, the article denounced the use of electrotherapy for war neurosis, which had soon emptied neurological clinics of their patients. It claimed that the pain inflicted by the treatment was so severe that many died and others fled from the hospitals to avoid torture. Wagner-Jauregg's Clinic was mentioned as one of the worst, and two further articles, published in February and March 1919 respectively, under the title 'Physicians or torturers?' gave fuller details. As a result of the agitation the provisional National Assembly on 19 December 1918 set up a Commission of five members to investigate derelictions of military duty. The Commission had no legal function, its sole purpose being to determine whether grounds existed for instituting a legal prosecution.

The Chairman was an eminent academic lawyer and the other members were two medical men (including Wagner-Jauregg), another lawyer and the editor of the *Arbeiterzeitung* (a Socialist daily). It began its work on 15 March 1919 and by June of the same year the Commission considered 164 cases. A complaint by one Walter Kauders was specifically aimed at Wagner-Jauregg's Clinic, and this meant that the case against Wagner-Jauregg had to be heard. As a result Wagner-Jauregg had to relinquish his function as a member of the Commission. The hearings of the case against him and other physicians took place on 14 and 16 October 1920, the findings of the Commission being reported on 24 October and published in the *Wiener Medizinische Wochenschrift*.[6]

The records of the Austrian proceedings have been studied and essential parts of them have been published with critical comments by K.R. Eissler.[7] The hearings began with an outline by the Chairman of the accusations brought against a number of physicians, which included severe damage through electrotherapy, solitary confinement and unpleasant medication. Wagner-Jauregg was called upon to comment on these accusations, particularly on the electrotherapy used at his Clinic. Speaking on war neuroses in general, he said that the most common symptom was that people were unable to walk. The number of such cases had reached epidemic proportions. Hysteria, Wagner-Jauregg said, was an infectious disease, and the peculiar neuroses involving movement were an epidemic caused by the war. It was the soldier's attitude to the war that determined whether he was likely to suffer from such a neurosis.

The principal expert witness on the first day of the proceedings was Freud (1856–1939). Although his biographer, Ernest Jones, believed that Freud had been called because of his scientific reputation[8], Eissler[9] thinks that his involvement was attributable to the difficulty experienced by the authorities (according to an article in the *Neue Freie Presse* of 29 May 1920) in finding experts to give evidence. Most of the specialists in the subject were followers, students or friends of Wagner-Jauregg, and the Commission was anxious not to be accused of a lack of objectivity. Also Freud was known to the Chairman who, in inviting Freud to give evidence, asked whether he was fundamentally opposed to Wagner-Jauregg and the Vienna School. Before Freud could answer, Wagner-Jauregg interjected, asking how this could be since he had never written anything on 'the subject'. (Presumably he meant psychoanalysis.) Freud, in reply, stated that he did not think there was an essential difference between himself and Wagner-Jauregg on the subject of war neuroses, except that he would have found fewer cases of simulation and more of neurosis. He was entirely convinced that his friend Wagner-Jauregg, whom he had known for thirty-five years and whose driving motive was the treatment of the sick, could not possibly be among those physicians who had forgotten their duty to humanity. Although certain that there was no question of a dereliction of duty, he believed that psychoanalysis would have proved more successful than the physical therapies adopted.

It is clear from Wagner-Jauregg's remarks in his *Memoirs*[10] that he was deeply hurt and found the proceedings painful. For a man in his position to be accused of inhumanity must have been traumatic, and this partly explains his somewhat unjustified comments about Freud's evidence being unfavourable. He thought that Freud had tried to vent his anger because of the attacks he had endured from Wagner-Jauregg's assistant, E. Raimann. Although the tension during the hearing emerges from the record of the proceedings – both Wagner-Jauregg and Freud sound touchy and irritable – a reading of the transcripts does not suggest that Freud said anything against Wagner-Jauregg. He seems, indeed, to have been at pains to stress that there could be no question of dereliction of duty on the part of Wagner-Jauregg.

On the second day of the hearing evidence was given by a number of medical experts, including three professors of psychiatry who were or had been assistants to Wagner-Jauregg. All witnesses joined in an attack against psychoanalysis and Freud who himself was not present that day. In a letter to K. Abraham (1877–1925) dated 31 October 1920,[11] Freud commented that these attacks against psychoanalysis showed the hatred the local psychiatrists felt towards him, and it was significant that they had occurred when he was not present. In his presence these witnesses pretended to be friendly.

In the report by the Commission, published on 24 October 1920[12], Wagner-Jauregg's work was praised and he was entirely exonerated from the accusations that had been levelled against him. The Commission did, however, come to the conclusion that Dr M. Kozlowski, one of Wagner-Jauregg's assistants, who had carried out most of the treatments of Faradism, seemed to have been largely responsible for the malpractices that had occurred. (He was no longer in Vienna and did not appear before the Commission.) He had acted against Wagner-Jauregg's instructions and applied the electrically charged brush not only to the extremities, but even to the testicles. Moreover, these treatments had been witnessed by onlookers who uttered derisive exclamations and threats. A number of witnesses gave damaging evidence against Kozlowski, but Wagner-Jauregg seemed to have been unaware of the malpractices of his assistant. This may seem difficult to credit, but in his critical comments Eissler stressed that, although Wagner-Jauregg was an outstanding medical man, he was no psychologist; he probably thought that Kozlowski was conscientious, and 'naivety is not unusual in great men.'[13]

Wagner-Jauregg's attitude to psychology is illustrated by an incident told by E. Stransky,[14] who later became one of his assistants. When examined by Wagner-Jauregg on Dementia senilis Stransky, in his reply, used words such as 'association' and 'apperception' which he had learned from studying Wundt's psychology.* Wagner-Jauregg interrupted him somewhat brusquely: 'What do you mean by these terms? Express yourself in a less affected manner!' Stransky substituted more commonly used terms and passed. According to him, Wagner-Jauregg was not in favour of experimental psychology and doubted its value for clinical work. He disliked the intrusion of complicated psychological terms into psychiatry and it is not surprising that psychoanalysis did not appeal to him.†

---

* Wilhelm Wundt (1832–1920).

† The general attitude to psychoanalysis in Viennese academic circles may be gleaned from a remark in the autobiography of Hilde Spiel[15] who was a student of psychology in the 1930s. She writes that she had read Freud's most important writings, but graduated in psychology in 1936 without ever having been asked about him.

FREUD AND WAGNER-JAUREGG

Freud and Wagner-Jauregg had been students together at the University of Vienna and at first their careers ran on similar lines. They were almost exact contemporaries, Freud having been born in 1856, Wagner-Jauregg in 1857. They got to know each other during their student days at the University of Vienna where they attended the same courses and for a short time worked together in Stricker's Institute for Experimental Pathology. In 1882 both Freud and Wagner-Jauregg applied for the position of assistant at H. Nothnagel's Clinic for Internal Medicine, but neither got the post. The father of the successful candidate had worked with Nothnagel in Berlin, an instance of how much personal influence mattered in medical circles. Whereas Wagner-Jauregg remained at Stricker's Institute, Freud, who was in financial difficulties, followed the advice of Ernst von Brücke, the Director of the Institute for Physiology where he had been working for six years, to abandon his scientific career. He therefore entered the General Hospital where he worked in different departments until the autumn of 1885 when he left for Paris to study under Charcot.

In 1884 Freud's and Wagner-Jauregg's paths crossed briefly. They both spent some of their spare time in Stricker's Institute and participated, with others, in animal experiments investigating the function of glands in relation to the circulatory system. During the same year they met to settle a priority dispute between Carl Koller and Leopold Königstein (1850–1924), both ophthalmologists. Freud had demonstrated the anaesthetising properties of cocaine to both. Koller and Königstein experimented successfully with its use in eye operations and reported on it to the Vienna Medical Society on 17 October 1884. However, Koller had already publicised his results a month earlier at the Ophthalmological Congress in Heidelberg. Freud recalls in a letter how he and Wagner-Jauregg were called upon to settle the dispute amicably, which they did by persuading Königstein to insert a letter in the *Wiener Medizinische Presse* to the effect that he conceded priority to Koller.[16]

In 1885 both Freud and Wagner-Jauregg were awarded the 'Dozentur' (the first step in an academic career in German-speaking countries)* in the field of neuropathology, which entitled them to give lectures at the University. This is usually granted on the strength of published work and a lecture. The application must be supported by

---

* *Venia legendi.*

members of the Professorial Board, and Freud's was supported by Brücke, Meynert and Nothnagel. It was granted by the Faculty by twenty-one votes to one, in view of the number of papers Freud had already to his credit. On the other hand, there was some opposition to the award of Wagner-Jauregg's Dozentur because of his inexperience. His application was supported by Leidesdorf, but opposed by Meynert, Leidesdorf's rival, who only changed his mind when pressed to do so by Stricker.[17]

Until then Freud's and Wagner-Jauregg's career had proceeded on similar lines, but from that time they went their different ways, and as far as is known met rarely. With their habilitation as 'Dozent' they were both entitled to give lectures at the University on neuropathology. Wagner-Jauregg had been fortunate in becoming an assistant in a psychiatric clinic where he was reasonably well paid, housed and fed. Soon after he joined the clinic, he was promoted and entered on his successful career as a psychiatrist. Freud, on the other hand, was working in the General Hospital at a very low salary and under conditions that compared unfavourably with those of Wagner-Jauregg. Moreover, Freud had become engaged in 1882 and was very anxious to marry and settle down.

Towards the end of February 1885 Freud was informed that his chief, F. Scholz, the Head of the Department for Nervous Diseases, wished him to be transferred to another department because it would seem that he had had some differences with his chief. Freud protested, but to no avail. Jones writes that Freud left Scholz's Department with regret, partly because he had to relinquish courses which he enjoyed giving and partly because he was deprived of the use of patients for teaching purposes.[18] He then spent some months in the Department of Ophthalmology and the Department of Dermatology before, in the autumn of that year, he was awarded a travel grant by the University which he proposed to use to study under Charcot in Paris. Although he could have had six months' leave of absence from the hospital, he chose to resign, arriving in Paris in October 1885 and attending the Salpêtrière for four months until March 1886.

On his return to Vienna Freud set up in practice and took over a new neurological department at the public Institute for Children's Diseases. He was, in addition, offered the facilities of Meynert's Clinic which were, however, withdrawn when Freud refused to rule out the use of hypnotism, and the arrangement came to an end. Freud complained that he had nowhere to deliver his lectures.[19]

On 15 October 1886 Freud presented a paper 'On male

hysteria' to the Vienna Medical Society in which he praised the work of Charcot and the achievements of the French school.[20] The lecture was not received with much enthusiasm, but from reading the report of the meeting it is difficult to understand why the reception of his lecture rankled with Freud for the rest of his life. However, the atmosphere of a meeting rarely emerges from a printed report and Freud's view is confirmed by Wagner-Jauregg. He wrote, 'Freud praised Charcot in enthusiastic terms which the Vienna celebrities could not abide. Bamberger and Meynert in the discussion bluntly rejected Freud's statements and thus he fell into disgrace with the Faculty.'[21]

Although as a Dozent Freud was entitled to give lectures – an opportunity which he made use of – he was never a regular academic teacher. The titles of 'Extraordinary Professor' awarded to him in 1902 and of 'Ordinary Professor' in 1919 were both purely *titular*, a fact that is omitted in most biographies. Wagner-Jauregg became an 'Extraordinary Professor' in 1889 and a full professor in 1893, only five and nine years respectively after his Habilitation, whereas Freud had to wait seventeen years for the one and thirty-four years for the other, and was then only awarded the titles.

Two historians of medicine, a husband-and-wife team, J. and R. Gicklhorn, investigated the reasons for Freud's slow and essentially unsatisfactory academic career and contrasted it with that of Wagner-Jauregg.[22 and 23] They maintained that Freud's lack of success in his academic career was entirely his own fault, in that, by refusing to accept the Dozentur in psychiatry, Freud damaged his academic career and impeded his promotion. K.R. Eissler has pointed out, however, that this is simply not true because a Dozentur must be applied for and Freud did not do this.[24] In any case, it is unlikely that Freud would have been successful in an application for Habilitation in psychiatry, since his work and his publications had been on neuroses which at the time were considered a specialised field only marginally related to psychiatry and had received only scant attention in contemporary textbooks. That this is the case is shown by a report by Wagner-Jauregg in 1899 to the Professorial Board on the selection of a candidate for a Chair, in which he stated that 'Dr Freud is only Dozent for neuropathology and has never really worked in psychiatry.'[25]

As far as can be ascertained, the facts regarding Freud's professorships are as follows. The Professorial Board in 1897 planned to appoint Freud to an extraordinary professorship, a proposal made by H. Nothnagel, Professor of Internal Medicine, and R. von Krafft-Ebing, Professor of Psychiatry. This and other recommendations for promotion were submitted to the Ministry of Education, but none was acceded to, probably for reasons of economy. However, in 1900, all the recommendations except that of Freud were approved. It was not until two influential patients of Freud's, Frau Elise Gomperz and Baroness Marie Ferstel, intervened and Nothnagel and Krafft-Ebing repeated their recommendations that the *title* of Extraordinary Professor was granted to Freud.[26]

J. Gicklhorn suggests that the title of Ordinary Professor which Freud received in 1919 was due to Wagner-Jauregg's initiative. It is true that Wagner-Jauregg wrote a favourable, if somewhat lukewarm, report on Freud's achievements at the request of the permanent Commission whose duty it was to make recommendations to the Medical Faculty on appointments and promotions. It seems, however, much more likely, as Eissler suggests, that the decision to award the title to Freud was due to the intervention of Otto Bauer, a friend of Freud's, who at the time was Foreign Minister.[27] This appointment too was purely titular. Freud described it as an 'empty title', since it brought with it no seat on the Board of the Faculty, nor did it bring any special teaching responsibilities.[28]

It is clear that Wagner-Jauregg did not wish to obstruct Freud's promotion, and although formally supporting it, he found difficulty in saying much in favour of Freud. Freud's theories, he wrote, even if they were not going to be upheld, contained many ingenious and valuable observations, not merely hypotheses, so that whether or not one agreed with them, recognition of Freud's work should not be denied.[29]

In his *Memoirs* Wagner-Jauregg wrote[30] that there had never been a dispute between them since he realised that Freud's theories brought new insights, although he believed that Freud was inclined to exaggerations and unfounded generalisations. Occasionally, among friends, but never in public, he had made harmless and humorous remarks about some of Freud's statements. This is confirmed in Paul Roazen's biography of Helene Deutsch.[31] 'Wagner-Jauregg,' he writes, 'may have made jokes about Freud, but he genuinely respected him as well; he did not consider him an advocate of dirty sex, as was common in Munich.' However, it is clear that he was critical of psychoanalysis and, according to Roazen, Wagner-Jauregg objected that Freud thought that analysis could do everything. He was more mocking than aggressively hostile, maintaining a tolerant but sarcastic attitude toward psychoanalysis. His scepticism was also a result of his fear that 'nonsense like psychoanalysis' could cause real harm. Stransky[32] wrote that Wagner-Jauregg used to say that psychoanalysis was not a scientific school, but a sect, in the theories of which one could believe or not. He did, however, admit that through Freud more attention was given to the psyche of nervous patients than before, which was to be welcomed. He recognised the need for a rational psychological treatment of neuroses and Freud's merits in this respect, but he had no liking for the schools of depth-psychology and denied them any curative value. According to Peter Berner,[33] one of the principal reasons for the scepticism of the descriptive school of psychiatry concerning psychoanalysis was a reticence towards generalizations. Wagner-Jauregg and his disciples recognised the psychological aspects of mental troubles and accepted the principle of the psycho-dynamic origin of neuroses, but remained sceptical towards doctrinal statements.

Although Wagner-Jauregg seems to have refrained from commenting openly on Freud and psychoanalysis, a confidential report that he submitted to the Professorial Board when Alfred Adler (1870–1937) applied for a Dozentur shows clearly what his opinion was.[34] In it he recommended that the Board ought to consider whether it was fitting for a representative of the psychoanalytical school to teach in the medical faculty of the University. Adler was under the influence of a theory which could not be surpassed in its 'hair-raising brutality'. In Adler's theory the sexual aspect played a similar role to that of Freud's. To give everything a sexual connotation Adler used a far-reaching symbolism which was no better than Freud's grotesque symbolism.

Nevertheless, although most of Wagner-Jauregg's assistants were antagonistic to psychoanalytic work, those who were in favour were allowed to carry on as they liked. Unlike Freud, Wagner-Jauregg was very tolerant and made allowances for different scientific opinions, even when they ran counter to his own. He allowed Freud's disciples, such as Schilder and Hartmann, to lecture on psychoanalysis, and – according to Anna Freud's biographer, Elisabeth Young-Bruehl – granted her permission to join the morning ward-rounds to gain some experience with psychiatric diagnosis, which she did for about a year.[35] Yet Freud found it difficult to believe that E. Raimann, Wagner-Jauregg's assistant, who was very much opposed to psychoanalysis and, as referee for psychiatric and psychological periodicals, had plenty of opportunity to pour scorn on Freud's publications, would speak as he did unless he had his chief's approval.

Despite their diametrically opposed scientific views, it does seem that Wagner-Jauregg and Freud had very friendly feelings for each other and used the familiar term 'Du' in their correspondence. One example is a reply to Wagner-Jauregg's congratulations on Freud's 60th birthday. In it he wrote:

> Your letter was one of the most pleasing which have reached me on the occasion of my sixtieth birthday. It assured me of your friendly sentiments which I would always have valued the more because we are going different ways in science. I must confess to you that until today I had not been sure of these. During the thirty years that we have been living in the same city as professional colleagues I have rarely experienced signs of your interest and in view of the unworthy treatment which my scientific writings have received by persons in your entourage, I have often been able to ask myself in what way such behaviour enjoys your approval. I therefore consider your lines as an unambiguous expression of your personal sentiment for which I thank you heartily and sincerely.[36]

Again there was an exchange of letters between the old colleagues on the occasion of Wagner-Jauregg's 75th birthday in 1932, when, in reply to a letter of congratulation from Freud and the Vienna Psychoanalytical Association, Wagner-Jauregg wrote:

> Dear Friend,
> Thank you sincerely for the friendly congratulations on my 75th birthday which you conveyed as Chairman of the Psychoanalytical Association as well as on your own behalf which pleases me specially. I take this opportunity to defend myself against the accusation of being an opponent of psychoanalysis. As far as I can remember, the first and only time I wrote about psychoanalysis was in the year 1930 in a newspaper article when reviewing a work by Alexander and Staub[37] on psychoanalysis in criminal law practice. I believe that whoever reads this article will not be able to claim that I acted as an opponent of psychoanalytic theory; I only claimed the right to criticise. For the psychoanalytic theory which you created is not a dogma which appeals to faith, but a scientific work which, despite its magnificence, may be criticised in its

particulars. For what one-time students of mine have written against psychoanalysis I take no responsibility. I only want to stress that others at my Clinic, I will only mention Poetzl, Schilder, Hartmann, have written approvingly of psycho-analytic theories without my taking it amiss. I therefore ask you to thank the members of the Psychoanalytical Association for their congratulations and to tell them that they should not consider me an opponent but an unprejudiced person who needs to be persuaded.

I am also particularly pleased that this occasion has brought me in personal touch with you and thus to be re-minded of a time already fifty years ago.[38]

It has been stated that the two old colleagues remembered each other on their 80th birthdays, but it has not been possible to confirm this.

REFERENCES

[1] Paul Roazen. *Helene Deutsch. A Psychoanalyst's Life*. New American Library, 1985.

[2] D. Langer. *Paul Ferdinand Schilder. Leben und Werk*. Thesis, Mainz, 1979.

[3] S.L. Last, 'Perspective'. *Psychiat.Bull.*, 1989, 13: p. 401.

[4] Julius Wagner-Jauregg. Erfahrungen über Kriegsneurosen. *Wien. Med.Wschr.*, 1916, 66: no. 36, 1355–8; no. 45, 1677–80; 1917, 67: no. 4, 189–93; no. 21, 929–33; 1918, 68: no. 43, 1877–83.

[5] Julius Wagner-Jauregg. *Lebenserinnerungen*. Ed. L. Schönbauer and M. Jantsch. Wien: Springer, 1950, p. 70.

[6] A. Löffler. Kommission zur Erhebung militärischer Pflichtver-letzungen. *Wien.Med.Wschr.*, 1920, 70: no. 46, 1951.

[7] K.R. Eissler. *Freud und Wagner-Jauregg vor der Kommission zur Erhebung militärischer Pflichtverletzungen*. Wien: Löcker Verlag, 1979; also transl by Christine Trollope under the title *Freud as an expert witness*. Madison, CT: International Universities Press, 1986.

[8] Ernest Jones. *Sigmund Freud. Life and work*. London: Hogarth Press, 1956–57, Volume III, p. 22.

[9] Eissler, op.cit. ref 7, p. 30.

[10] Wagner-Jauregg, op.cit. ref 5, p. 73.

[11] Hilda Abraham and E.L. Freud, ed. *A Psychoanalytic Dialogue: The letters of Sigmund Freud and Karl Abraham, 1907–1926*. London: Hogarth Press, 1965, p. 317.

[12] Löffler, op.cit. ref 6.

[13] Eissler, op.cit. ref 7, p. 104.

[14] E.S. Stransky. *Selbstbiographie*. M.S. held at the Institut für Geschichte der Medizin der Universität Wien.

[15] Hilde Spiel. *Die hellen und die finsteren Zeiten. Erinnerungen 1911–1946*. München: List Verlag, 1989, p. 133.

[16] Leopold Königstein. *Wien.Med.Presse*, 1884, nos. 42 and 43.

[17] Wagner-Jauregg, op.cit. ref 5, pp. 43–44.

[18] Jones, op.cit. ref 8, Vol. I, p. 81.

[19] Ibid. pp. 257–8.

[20] Sigmund Freud. Ueber männliche Hysterie. *Wien.Med.Wschr.*, 1886, 34: no. 43, 1444–47.

[21] Wagner-Jauregg, op.cit. ref 5, p. 72.

[22] J. Gicklhorn. Julius Wagner-Jaureggs Gutachten über Sigmund Freud und seine Studien zur Psychoanalyse. *Wien.Klin.Wschr.*, 1957, 69: no. 30, 533–537.

[23] J. and R. Gicklhorn. *Sigmund Freuds akademische Laufbahn*. Wien und Innsbruck: Urban und Schwarzenberg, 1960.

[24] K.R. Eissler. Julius Wagner-Jaureggs Gutachten über Sigmund Freud und seine Studien zur Psychoanalyse. *Wien.Klin.Wschr.*, 1958, 70: no. 22, 402; *Sigmund Freud und die Wiener Universität*. Bern und Stutgart: Huber, 1966.

[25] Eissler, ibid. p. 64.

[26] Jones, op.cit. ref 8, Vol. I, pp. 373–374.

[27] Eissler, op.cit. ref 24.

[28] Jones, op.cit. ref 8, Vol. III, p. 18.

[29] Eissler, op.cit. ref 24.

[30] Wagner-Jauregg, op.cit. ref 5, p. 73.

[31] Roazen, op.cit. ref 1, p. 116.

[32] Stransky, op.cit. ref 14.

[33] Peter Berner. La psychiatrie Viennoise entre Freud et Wagner von Jauregg. *Bull.Acad.Nat.Med.*, 1988, 172: no. 2, 191–195.

[34] MS held at the University Archives, University of Vienna.

[35] Elisabeth Young-Bruehl. *Anna Freud. A biography*. New York: Summit Books, 1988.

[36] L. Schönbauer und M. Jantsch. Julius Wagner-Jauregg. In K. Kolle, ed. *Grosse Nervenärzte*. Stuttgart: Georg Thieme, 1956, pp. 254–266.

[37] F. Alexander und H. Staub. Der Verbrecher und seine Richter. Wien: 1929.

[38] Ibid.

ILLUSTRATIONS

---

1. Wagner-Jauregg *(Page v)*

2. Introduction from Wagner-Jauregg's *Memoirs* with translation and note
    (Pages vi and vii)

3. Wagner-Jauregg

4. Wagner-Jauregg and his son

5. Wagner-Jauregg

6. Bust of Wagner-Jauregg

7. Lecture Hall of the Second Psychiatric Clinic

8. The Vienna Asylum

9. and 10. Wagner-Jauregg's school

11. Plaque on the house where Wagner-Jauregg spent most of his adult life

12. Wagner-Jauregg with his disciples

13. Malaria blood sampling

14. Lecture Hall at the Institute for General and Experimental Pathology

15. Salomon Stricker

16. Richard von Krafft-Ebing

17. Maximilian Leidesdorf

18. Theodor Meynert

19. 500 Schilling note

20. 50 Schilling note

21. 2.40 Schilling stamp

22. 3 Schilling stamp

23. Wagner-Jauregg

24. Karl Stürgk

25. Alexander Girardi

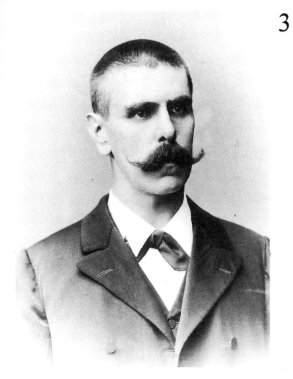

3

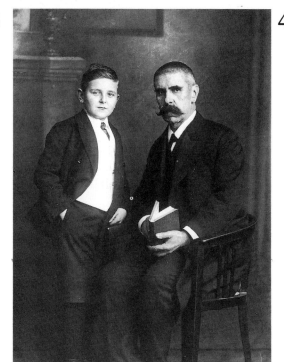

4

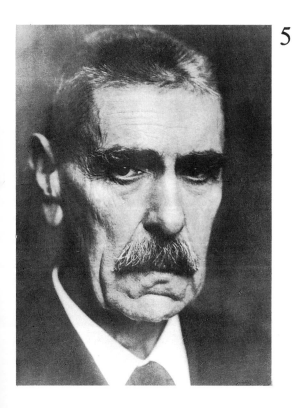

5

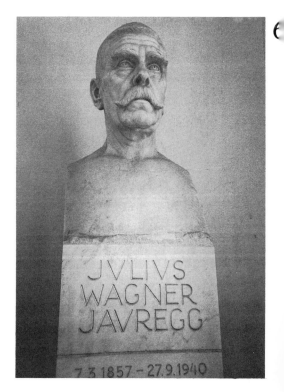

6

7

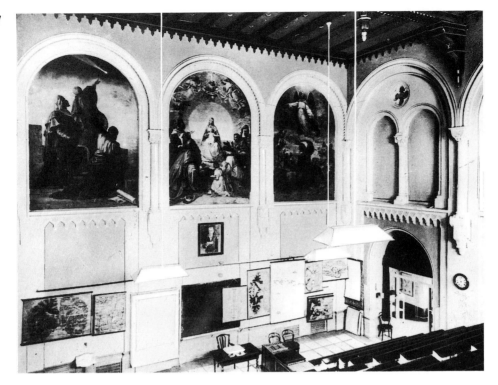

8

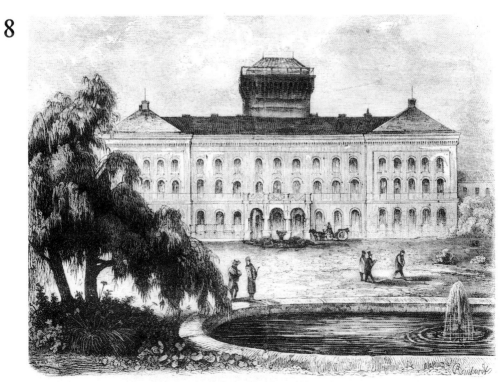

Die f. f. Irrenanstalt in Wien.

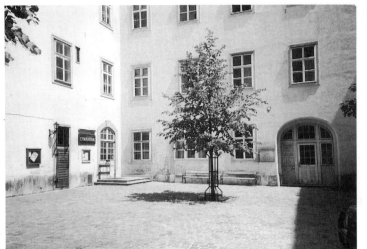

9

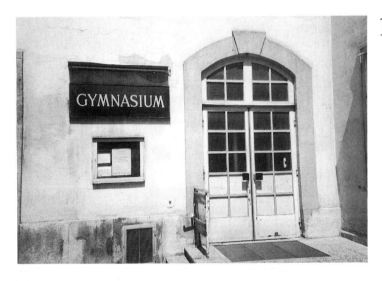

10

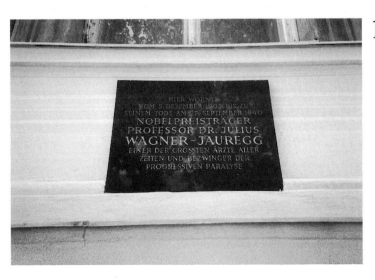

11

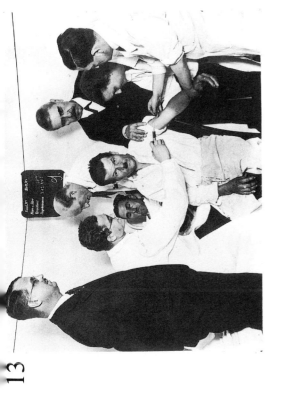

12

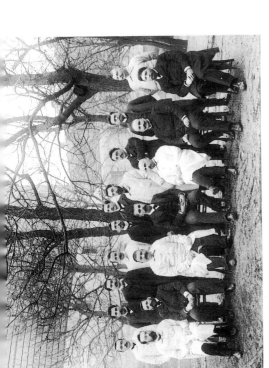

13

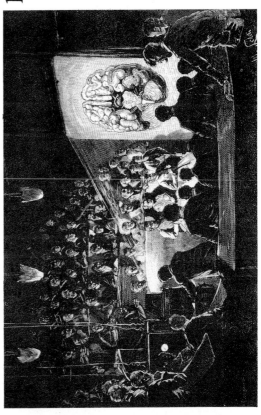

14

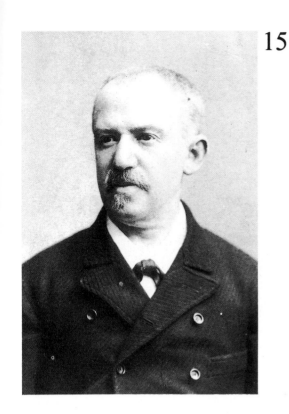

15

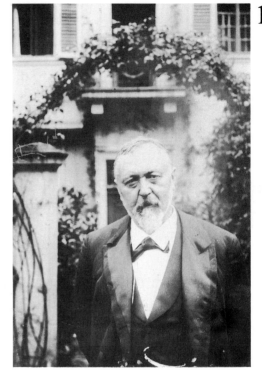

16

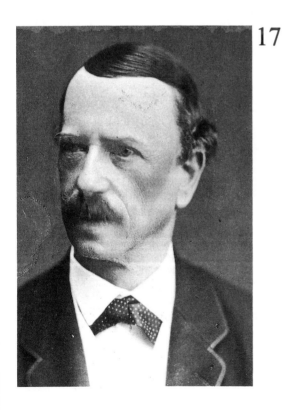

17

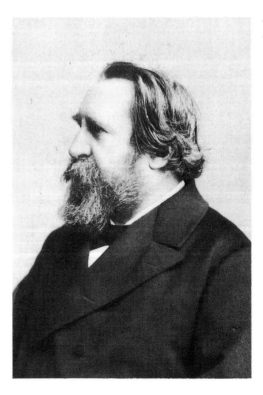

18

9

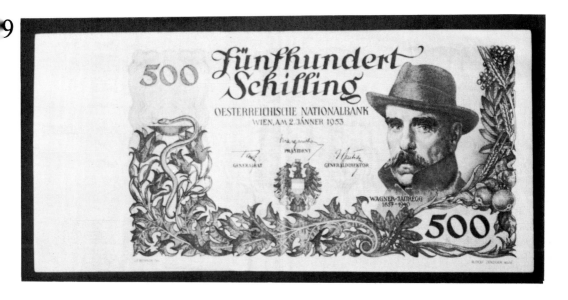

0

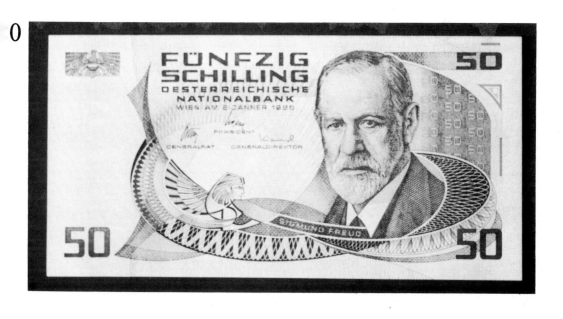

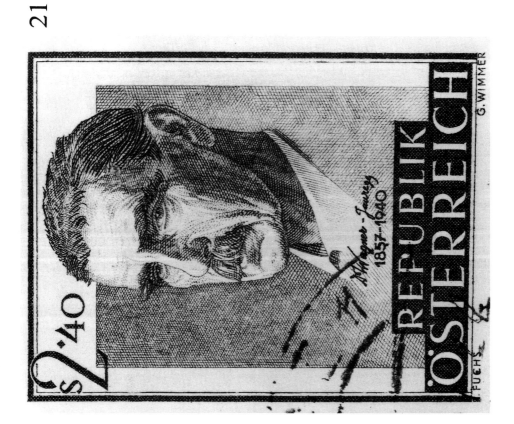

SIGMUND FREUD

REPUBLIK ÖSTERREICH

K. LEITGEB

A. PILCH

1856·1939

S 3

REPUBLIK ÖSTERREICH

G. WIMMER

1857–1940

J. FUCHS

2·40

23

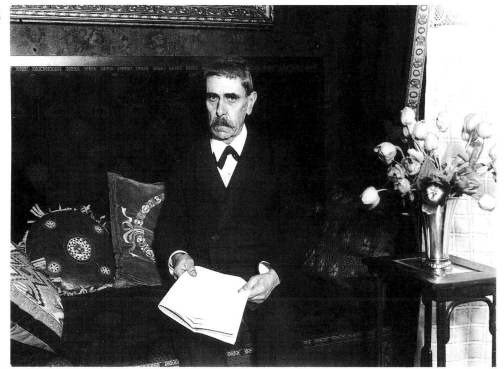

24

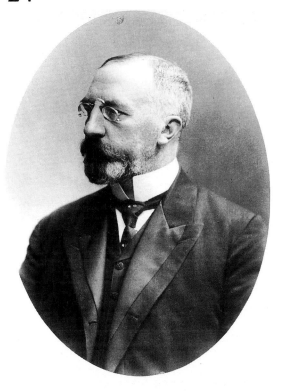

25

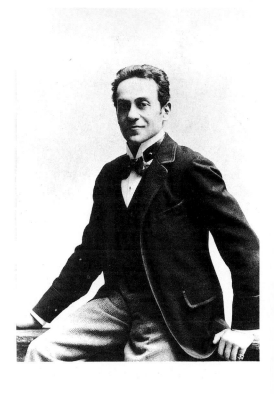

EIGHT

Wagner-Jauregg's Contribution to the Study of Cretinism

As related in the chapter on Wagner-Jauregg's activities in Graz, his friend Moritz Holl persuaded him to look into the problem of cretinism. He did not need much persuasion because he was greatly disturbed by the number of cretins they met on their mountain tours and because he had already taken up the subject when, in 1884, at the suggestion of his chief, Leidesdorf, he had carried out some experiments on animals on the effect of removing the thyroid gland. The reasons that led to Leidesdorf's suggestion were the reports from Swiss surgeons that patients who had their thyroid removed showed all the symptoms of cretinism. Developments in anaesthesia and asepsis had made goitre excisions a safe and much practised operation, but soon the consequences of thyroid excision became alarming. Accordingly, J.L. Reverdin (1842–1929)[1] modified his practice and removed only part of the thyroid. Th. Kocher (1841–1917) also discovered the adverse effects of the removal of the gland.[2] He found that, whereas those who only had part of the gland removed were in good health, those who had undergone total excision were in poor health, showing lassitude, weakness, feeling of cold, reduced mental alertness, slowness of speech and – in the case of juveniles – reduced growth. He called the syndrome *Cachexia strumipriva* and concluded that for the first time the relation between thyroid and cretinism had been established.

WAGNER-JAUREGG'S EXPERIMENTS

Wagner-Jauregg operated on eight cats and two dogs. One cat and one dog survived, both having only had one side of the thyroid removed. The others developed lassitude, convulsions and tetany, and died soon after the operation. In his *Memoirs*[3] Wagner-Jauregg recounts how he packed three of the cats on which he had operated in a bag and went to a meeting of the Vienna Medical Society. There he put the three cats on a table where they performed in the way he had predicted. Billroth, the Professor of Surgery, who was presiding, did not seem pleased as, at the time, he was seeking for another explanation of the behaviour of the animals. The Minutes of the meeting of the Vienna Medical Society on 13 June 1884 confirm Wagner-Jauregg's account. Billroth denied that goitre resections had any ill effect,[4] but it was known in Vienna that his patients had suffered effects similar to those observed by the Swiss surgeons.

Wagner-Jauregg's results of his experiments were published in a Vienna medical periodical in 1884.[5] As so often happens in the history of science, several workers embarked on similar experiments in the same year. One of them – the physiologist Moritz Schiff (1823–1926) from Geneva – extracted the thyroid gland from animals – mostly dogs – and observed symptoms which agreed entirely with those described by Wagner-Jauregg.[6] Neither knew of the other's experiments at the time, though subsequently they corresponded. Strangely, in all the accounts of these developments, Wagner-Jauregg's name has been omitted, yet he claimed in his *Memoirs*[7] to have been nearer the correct interpretation of the results than Schiff had been.

Wagner-Jauregg drew an analogy with the removal of both kidneys: the resection of only one side of the thyroid gland, just as the resection of only one kidney, led to the hypertrophy of the remaining part. The removal of both kidneys caused nervous symptoms and uraemia due to the accumulation of poisonous substances which collect in the blood; and similarly, Wagner-Jauregg claimed, since the thyroid plays a part in the body's metabolism, when its activity ceases certain substances accumulate which have a deleterious effect on the organism. This explained why, although the animals felt well immediately after the operation, later they gradually showed symptoms of disease. When, however, only part of the thyroid was removed, no deleterious effects resulted. Schiff, on the other hand, had furnished an incorrect explanation of the results of the removal, because he thought that there was a relation between the thyroid and the nutrition of the central nervous system.

Although Wagner-Jauregg continued with his research on the thyroid for some time, he eventually dropped the subject for a number of years. Later it transpired that neither he nor Schiff had realised that they had removed not only the thyroid gland but also the parathyroid glands. These had been discovered in 1880 by Ivar Sandström (1852–89), but he had published his results in a Swedish periodical and the news only reached Central Europe much later.[8] It proved that tetany, the lethal result of thyroidectomy, only occurred if the parathyroid glands were resected as well.

CRETINISM IN STYRIA

When in 1892 Wagner-Jauregg resumed his researches into the role of the thyroid in cretinism, he approached the problem from a different angle. He knew from experience that no cretins were ever brought to the Psychiatric Clinic. Occasionally they were seen at other clinics when they were ill or needed surgery, but never at the Psychiatric Clinic, despite their mental handicap, because they caused no trouble and were not dangerous. Moreover, it was well known that there was no cure for them.

Since the cretins did not come to the Clinic, Wagner-Jauregg went to look for them in the countryside and in his *Memoirs* he gave a vivid account of his researches. He chose as his field of investigation the district of Frohnleiten, which was easily accessible from Graz. He procured a list of the mentally sick, the cretins and the deaf-mutes in private care in the district, which, according to the health regulations then in force, had to be kept by the chief magistrate. He also asked the local authorities at Graz for permission to make investigations, and he was given a document with which to establish his identity. He found it easy to gain access to hundreds of households and only twice was he given an unfriendly welcome by a mother who would not admit that one of her offspring was 'not quite right in the head'. Generally, the document made the desired impression, particularly, Wagner-Jauregg commented, because the peasants were not very good at reading.

Throughout the summer months of 1892 Wagner-Jauregg spent every Thursday afternoon and Sunday in search of cretins. This was a strenuous activity because he was on his feet all the time, climbing mountains and wandering through valleys. The communities covered a large area, the difference in height between them being often up to 800 metres, which explains why in the district of Frohnleiten he was only able to visit nine of the fourteen communities. Often there was no opportunity for him to have a proper lunch. Usually, he went first to the local offices of the parish or town to look through the lists of mentally handicapped and then visited them in their homes. He also made enquiries of people he met whether they knew of any other mentally handicapped individuals in their neighbourhood. In this way he found many more than appeared on the official lists and also soon realised that the distinctions between cretins, imbeciles and deaf-mutes on these lists were unreliable.

Wagner-Jauregg spent a few days in another district in Styria in which, according to official statistics, there were more cretins than in any other part of Austria. He did not go to the different houses, but asked the district medical officer to bring the cases to him in the district office. He was greatly surprised when he found that five or six times as many as the total number on the lists presented themselves. Later that year he made an expedition for the same purpose to another district of Styria where he was able to join the district medical officer on his tour of inspection. Wagner-Jauregg was particularly interested to discover how the incidence of cretinism changed after the river Mur left the mountains and was flowing through the plain. As he expected, cretinism disappeared there except for a few cases.

In connection with these investigations Wagner-Jauregg made a statistical study of cretinism, and of the way in which evidence was collected in Austria relating to the mentally ill, cretins and deaf-mutes in private care; he suggested ways of improving these methods. Two lengthy papers appeared in the *Jahrbücher für Psychiatrie* for 1893 and 1894 respectively.[10] In them he analysed the tables showing the numbers of cretins, deaf-mutes and mentally deficient during the years 1873–1890 in Styria, but found that they did not give a true picture of the situation. According to these statistics, the number of cretins increased with age, although one would expect the largest number to be among the younger age groups. Wagner-Jauregg believed that this discrepancy was due to faulty classification, since the returns were made by council officials who were not medically trained and thus unable to decide whether an individual was a cretin or was suffering from some other form of mental deficiency. He found that the classification into the three categories – cretins, insane and deaf-mutes – was often wrong, suspecting that the figures for deaf-mutes included cretins and other mentally deficient persons. In areas in which there were cretins, the number of deaf-mutes was considerable, because all cretins, to a greater or lesser degree, were hard of hearing, and those with not very clear cretinous symptoms tended to be classed among the deaf-mutes.

Wagner-Jauregg tried to make use of the schools for obtaining better statistics. The principal of each school received particulars of all the children in his district who were of school age, including those who were ineducable because they were mentally handicapped or were deaf-mutes. He therefore sent questionnaires to the school administrators of one district in Styria, but found the results to be unreliable. Also, at his request, the School Council for Styria made enquiries of all schools in that province to elicit the number of children of school age and the number of mentally deficient children for all twenty districts.

Wagner-Jauregg made a number of suggestions for obtaining more reliable statistics. The compilation of registers giving full details of the cretins, the mentally sick and the deaf-mutes should be made obligatory for all councils, and should be checked and updated each year. He emphasised the importance of calling upon medical experts to decide who should be classed as cretins.

DIFFICULTY IN DIAGNOSING CRETINISM

However, at the time even experienced physicians still had great difficulty in distinguishing between different forms of what was then termed imbecility or idiocy, and standard classifications made no distinction. It was the mongolian type that presented the greatest difficulty because mongols bore a close resemblance to cretins, although they showed no myxoedema.

In an extensive lecture to the Medical Society of Styria in March 1893 Wagner-Jauregg described the most important characteristics of a cretin.[11] The growth of cretins was stunted – dwarf-like in extreme cases and much below average in moderate cases – although at birth there was no difference from normal children. Cretins were seldom slender, like other imbeciles, but on the plump side. Their physiognomy was very distinctive owing to a shortening in the base of the skull which may be recognised by the shape of the nose, the root of which was drawn in, the wings being broad and shortened. The soft parts showed swellings of the skin and tissues, a thickening of the skin of the head, forehead, the lids and other parts of the body, typical of the symptoms of myxoedema. Another characteristic of cretins was the stunted development of the genitalia. Apart from the reduced physical development, the mental development of cretin was extremely slow, particularly in acquiring the ability to speak and to walk. One of the most important symptoms of cretinism was goitre. Endemic cretinism and endemic goitre usually occurred together, and those cretins who had no goitre were found to have no thyroid.

CRETINISM DUE TO MALFUNCTION OF THE THYROID

Summing up his findings, Wagner-Jauregg claimed that the phenomenon of cretinism could be explained, without exception, by the malfunction of the thyroid gland, a view that was supported by Th. Kocher[12], who had found that sporadic cretinism resulted from the total resection of goitre in young persons. Wagner-Jauregg's lecture was published in the *Communications of the Medical Society of Styria*, a periodical which unfortunately was not widely distributed. Consequently, his theory remained largely unknown. Meanwhile Kocher had put forward the same theory independently of Wagner-Jauregg, but since he published it in a widely distributed journal, he was generally cited as its originator. Wagner-Jauregg believed, however, that his version of the theory had more merit than Kocher's. The latter had blamed a brain defect for the speech impediment of cretins and had treated the endemic deaf-mutism as a separate matter, the consequence of a sense defect, whereas Wagner-Jauregg had been able to show that the majority of cretins suffered from definite auditory disturbances and that their inability to speak or to articulate properly – their language consisting of vowels and diphthongs only – was occasioned by their deafness. Learning to speak was a matter of imitating heard sounds. If hearing was impaired, then a proper imitation of sounds could not take place. Since the sound content of consonants was much less than that of vowels and diphthongs, the inability of cretins to speak properly became comprehensible.

Following Wagner-Jauregg's move from Graz to Vienna, the problem of cretinism receded into the background of his work for a few years, but in 1896 or 1897 (later he could not remember exactly when) he once again took up the problem. One of his colleagues referred to him a case of sporadic cretinism – an idiot child, retarded in growth and development, with thick tongue, hardly able to speak. Wagner-Jauregg already knew that in such cases the thyroid gland was missing. He was well informed in foreign literature and he was aware that in England physicians had already begun to treat such children successfully with fresh thyroid extract from sheep. He, therefore, began to use such a therapy on this girl and soon noticed a distinct improvement. He continued to treat her for several years, but soon substituted thyroid tablets for the thyroid extract. In the course of a few years this previously completely cretinous child developed into a normal woman who could almost be described as pretty. She attended primary school, learned to speak French and to play the piano, although she remained somewhat childish and was never self-reliant. Wagner-Jauregg lost sight of her later and did not know whether she eventually improved in that respect too. The case caused quite a stir and consequently a number of such cases were sent to him for treatment.[13]

WAGNER-JAUREGG'S THYROIDAL THEORY

As regards endemic cretinism, two interpretations had been put forward. According to that adopted by Kocher[14] and Wagner-Jauregg, it was simply infantile myxoedema, and all its symptoms, including imbecility, were due to the non-functioning of the thyroid. In the other interpretation, maintained by the Swiss surgeon H. Bircher (1850–1923)[15] and by the German physician C.A. Ewald (1845–1915)[16], the whole organism was diseased, particularly the brain, and the disease of the thyroid was only part of the syndrome.*

In his survey Wagner-Jauregg discussed in detail the most important symptoms of endemic cretinism to examine whether they could be explained by his theory. Since it had been established that goitrous degeneration of the thyroid could impair its function as could its atrophy, it was clear that goitre and cretinism were related. Ewald too had no doubt about this, but he believed, unlike Wagner-Jauregg, that the symptoms differed in endemic and sporadic

---

* Strangely in his *Memoirs* Wagner-Jauregg referred to both Kocher and Ewald as having contested his theory. Surely he must have meant Bircher not Kocher.[17]

cretinism. Bircher, on the other hand, argued that no change in thyroid function had been proved in cretinism and could not be considered as the cause of the disease.

In France, D.M. Bourneville (1840–1909)[18], who had made a study of sporadic cretinism, which he ascribed to athyroidism, refused to attribute endemic cretinism to the same cause. On the other hand, English physicians had recognised the identity of sporadic and endemic cretinism with infantile myxoedema. The first to take that point of view was F. Semon (1849–1921)[19], later adopted by all English researchers, most recently by G.R. Murray (1865–1939)[20].

THYROID THERAPY

The successes achieved in many countries, particularly in England, by injecting thyroid extract and administering thyroid tablets were remarkable. Myxoedema disappeared very quickly – within the first weeks, often within days, of beginning the therapy. Growth in height, in some cases considerable, was reported from America, England and Belgium. Wagner-Jauregg[21] treated a girl of 11, who had hardly grown for some time and was only 96 cm tall, but who after continuous treatment with thyroid extract and tablets for five years attained a height of 132 cm. Even in cases where normal growth had ceased, some patients in their twenties and thirties grew taller. The fontanelles, which in cretins remain open, closed up, and tooth and sexual development accelerated. As far as mental and nervous functions were concerned, successes were spectacular, but less so regarding intellectual development. This was not surprising since most of the cretins who had been treated were over ten years old, some even in their twenties and thirties, and their brains must have been damaged by the disease. However, reports of cretinous children under ten who were subjected to treatment were most encouraging. The paediatrician John Thomson (1856–1926) reported the case of a five-year-old girl who, after treatment, was able to attend school when she was eight with results comparable with those of healthy children.[22] A cretin before treatment could be described as a creature who in his deformity and ugliness not only elicited compassion but often repulsion, but who after treatment turned into a normal, and sometimes even a good-looking human being. In Wagner-Jauregg's view it was essential to continue the treatment throughout life, at first by giving large doses until the damage caused by athyroidism was remedied and then by reduced doses to maintain the improvement. Obviously, the sooner the treatment was begun the better. The difficulty was that cretinism at a very early age was difficult to diagnose. Murray,[23] therefore, recommended that, in the case of children who were slow to develop, thyroid tablets should be given for a few months as a trial. If development improved, this could be considered proof that the retarded development was due to athyroidism and that treatment should continue.

Wagner-Jauregg advised that such trials should be made extensively in the case of endemic cretinism. In view of the circumstances in which the victims of endemic cretinism were living, such trials would have to be organised by the central health authority. The importance of the matter was clear, if it was borne in mind that endemic cretinism in alpine countries and also in parts of Hungary and Galicia was a disease which claimed more victims than any other, except tuberculosis and syphilis.

ORGANISATION OF THYROID THERAPY IN STYRIA

Wagner-Jauregg then took practical steps to ensure that the treatment of cretins should be organised by the Government. He put his proposal before the Senior Health Council which accepted it unanimously.[24] He submitted concrete suggestions for treating cretins at as early an age as possible. The Civil Servant in charge, Dr Emanuel Kusy Ritter von Dubrav (1844–1905), who was on good terms with Wagner-Jauregg, proceeded to take action, but since, as Wagner-Jauregg remarked, he was a bureaucrat rather than a practitioner, he began to draw up documents for submission to the provincial governments which in their turn tried to shift responsibility on to the shoulders of others. The difficulty seems to have been the delicate relationship between central and provincial governments, both being anxious to retain their powers. Therefore the central government had to proceed gingerly to get anything done. Dr Kusy approached the Councils of Styria and Lower Austria suggesting that they should institute trials to fight cretinism, and he requested the pharmaceutical department of the General Hospital to supply Wagner-Jauregg with thyroid preparations without charge.

Wagner-Jauregg, realising that cretinism could not be cured

with ink, wondered what he could do himself to come to the aid of child cretins. Unexpectedly, he received help through the press, of which he usually had nothing good to say. Several newspapers, particularly in Styria, had reported his proposal to the Senior Health Council. As a result, a watchmaker in Judenburg, a small spa in Styria, who had three cretinous children, wrote to Wagner-Jauregg asking whether he thought that they would benefit from treatment. So Wagner-Jauregg travelled to Judenburg on 8 December 1900, examined the children and provided thyroid tablets from Burroughs Wellcome in London for the children to take.[25] He promised their father that he would return every three months to supervise the treatment and asked him to be on the look-out for child cretins whose parents were willing for them to be treated.

Wagner-Jauregg's request to the watchmaker was very successful. On his next visit he received information of other cases and from the relatives of these he was supplied with further addresses. Thus his circle of patients increased so much that he could no longer fit in all his visits on Sundays between fast trains to and from Vienna. Unfortunately, he found that doctors in Judenburg were not interested; they seemed indifferent, sometimes even antagonistic. Having visited Judenburg six or seven times, he thought of giving his attention to other places in the district where he knew cretinism to be endemic. Since he needed someone to direct him to child cretins, he approached the heads of schools (he thought they were more likely to help than doctors, after his experience at Judenburg), who were bound to know the cretins of school age. This aroused the professional ambition of three doctors in these places, and they communicated their interest and their willingness to help Wagner-Jauregg. They were two company doctors and one general practitioner. In one of these small towns there was no doctor, but the local head-master was willing to help. This programme was begun in August 1902, when Wagner-Jauregg took quarters in Judenburg and from there visited the other places.

He had particular success in one of the towns where he befriended the works doctor, R. Diviak, who, when he became convinced of the value of the treatment, pursued the matter with great zeal. Through him Wagner-Jauregg met the director of the rolling mill, who exerted influence on the relatives of the children that were being treated, to make sure that those children attended for examination and took the tablets regularly. The examinations, which usually took place three or four times a year, were attended by the otologist Gustav Alexander (1873–1932) from Vienna, who was interested in the hearing disorders of cretins and thus encouraged the whole enterprise. The tablets were placed at Wagner-Jauregg's disposal by order of Dr Kusy through Burroughs Wellcome in London; later they were produced by the Austrian State monopoly, but finally it was found cheaper to obtain them from Parke-Davis in London.

Thus Wagner-Jauregg embarked on a campaign of action which he continued until the outbreak of the First World War. It caused him a great deal of work and took up much of his free time, but he enjoyed it because it brought him out into the country and put him in touch with colleagues and people of all kinds. Above all it gave him great satisfaction to see imbecile children develop into normal human beings.

The Scholz affair

When the successful results of treatments in Judenburg became known the Professor of Internal Medicine at Graz University, Professor F. Kraus (1858–1936), instructed one of his assistants, Wilhelm Scholz (b. 1864) to carry out trials with thyroid therapy. This led to an unhappy experience for Wagner-Jauregg. Dr Scholz, who had not made a study of cretinism, armed himself with a large quantity of thyroid tablets and went to a hospital in a small town not far from Graz and there, with the permission of the medical superintendent, fed the pills to a number of cretins (Wagner-Jauregg suspected that among these were some non-cretinous imbeciles). At a congress on internal medicine, held in Graz in 1902, Scholz gave a talk in which (according to an account published in the *Wiener Klinische Wochenschrift*[26]) he reported on unsatisfactory results in the treatment of child cretins with thyroid preparations. There had been no growth in bone structure and, although no symptoms of poisoning were observed, there was considerable weakness and an increase in mental apathy. Wagner-Jauregg was not only greatly surprised, since these results were quite contrary to those he had for many years, but also very annoyed because he feared that Scholz's report could discredit his campaign both with the doctors and the population. Within three weeks he published in the same journal a short paper in which he described the great success he had in treating cretins with tablets from Burroughs Wellcome.[27] He thought that Scholz was quite wrong, and he was anxious that efforts at reducing cretinism should not be adversely affected. He left it to Scholz to find out the mistake he had made. Scholz completely ignored Wagner-Jauregg's comments and had his lecture published without any amendments. Wagner-Jauregg then took it on himself to find out what had gone wrong with Scholz's treatment. He thought at first that perhaps Scholz had used some ineffective medication, and so he went to the hospital where Scholz had made his trials and spoke to the medical superintendent. In the meantime, the one who had given permission for the trials to be carried out had died and his successor happened to be an old student of Wagner-Jauregg from his Graz days. With his help, Wagner-Jauregg discovered that the tablets used by Scholz were the same as he had prescribed, but the dosages were much larger. Wagner-Jauregg usually prescribed one tablet a day, and only in exceptional cases one and a half or two, and then never for long. Scholz, although he began with one tablet, had increased the dosage up to six tablets daily, which would account for his adverse results.[28]

Wagner-Jauregg published the results of his investigations in a short article in the *Communications of the Medical Society of Styria* in November 1903[29], hoping that Scholz would admit his mistake and the matter might thus be closed. But this was not the case: in a short note following Wagner-Jauregg's article Scholz denied ever having used more than three tablets a day, and moreover reiterated his statement that the tablets were not beneficial but injurious. So Wagner-Jauregg decided to investigate the matter further. Once again he went to see the medical superintendent of the hospital, who called the ward sister. She produced a piece of paper on which were written the names of the patients treated and, in each case, the dosage entered in Dr Scholz's handwriting: the dosage was six tablets. Moreover, the sister told Wagner-Jauregg that originally Scholz's idea was to increase the dosage to ten tablets, but as there had been three deaths following the treatment with six tablets, the medical superintendent would not allow the trials to continue. Although Wagner-Jauregg refused to take the document with him, as he considered it an important one which belonged to the hospital, he asked the medical superintendent to take good care of it, since it might be required as evidence. Nevertheless, when he returned to the hospital he was told that Scholz had been allowed to take the paper away with him.[30]

To Wagner-Jauregg's great satisfaction Scholz was punished

for his misconduct. At the Annual General Meeting of the German Society for Internal Medicine in Munich in April 1906, Professor Kraus who had instructed Scholz to make the trials was to give one of the two main reports on the pathology of the thyroid. Wagner-Jauregg expected him to try to justify Scholz's actions, and he therefore decided to attend the meeting, which he did not normally do. Professor Kraus – probably realising that he did not have a leg to stand on and that several workers had given good reports of the thyroid treatment of cretins – commented favourably on Wagner-Jauregg's work and said that his generously planned therapeutic enterprise to combat endemic cretinism by feeding cretins thyroid extracts had aroused interest. (A compliment that sounds somewhat lukewarm!) Consequently there was no discussion on the matter and moreover, Wagner-Jauregg had the satisfaction of seeing Scholz, who was sitting immediately in front of him, turn scarlet.[31]

RESULTS OF THYROID THERAPY

Wagner-Jauregg wrote two lengthy accounts of the treatment of endemic cretinism with thyroid preparations which were published in 1904 and 1907 respectively.[32] The first was based on a report submitted to the Ministry of the Interior on his activities in Styria in 1902 and 1903. He gave statistics on the increase in body height and quoted many cases in which considerable improvements occurred as a result of the treatment. The children got slimmer, although their appetite increased; they got livelier and moved better and their speech and hearing improved. Burroughs Wellcome had supplied tablets without charge; at first 10 000, and later many more. In the second report several more cases were described. Great improvements in the condition of the child cretins were achieved even when treatment was delayed, provided that it was not too late.

Wagner-Jauregg through his personal connections persuaded the Governor of Styria, who was a relative of his, to begin a campaign for the treatment of cretins in some districts of Upper Styria. He instructed the sanitary inspector at the Government Office, Dr Kutschera, to take the necessary measures. Kutschera, who had originally viewed the fight against cretinism with some scepticism, devoted himself to the campaign, which he began in 1905, with great enthusiasm.[33] He took care of all the districts visited by Wagner-

Jauregg, who was so pleased with his work that after 1908 he left all of them, except one, entirely to Kutschera.

Among Wagner-Jauregg's recently discovered papers is an incomplete draft[34] of a submission to the Health Department of the Ministry of the Interior in which he refers to a report by Dr Kutschera, which the Health Department allowed him to see, including photographs of 218 cretins and accounts of the favourable results achieved in treating over 700 children. Wagner-Jauregg urges publicity among the population and among doctors to alert them to the benefit of the treatment which he has been advocating and entreats the Health Department to further the endeavours of the Styrian Inspectorate.

Wagner-Jauregg took the opportunity to revert to a proposal he had made previously to permit a better evaluation of the treatment of cretins. It would be necessary to gain experience in the correct dosage of the medication at different stages of the treatment and at different ages. This would only be possible in an institution. The establishment and maintenance of such an institution, which need not be very large, was possible because a capital sum had become available in the so-called Cretinism Fund, the interest on which was being used not for the intended purpose, but towards the maintenance of an already existing institution for imbeciles, among whom there were no cretins. Wagner-Jauregg urges the Ministry to take steps to see that the Fund revert to its real purpose, the creation and maintenance of an institution for the study of cretinism. This had been advocated by the Minister, Graf Clary, for some time.

The manuscript is undated, but since Wagner-Jauregg refers in it to a paper of his which appeared in 1907 and to Dr Kutschera, who left the Styrian inspectorate in 1910 (he was appointed in that year Chief Inspector of Tirol and Vorarlberg, where he organised a similar campaign for the fight against cretinism), it must have been written between those two dates. The only other references so far discovered to the Institution described in the manuscript are in two obituaries of Wagner-Jauregg[35] which mention 'an institution in Zeltweg in Styria, established by Wagner-Jauregg with his own means in order to treat cretins systematically and to cure them, but which unfortunately had to close its doors during the difficult times after the First World War.'*

---

* Efforts to discover details of this Institution from the Styrian Archives have so far not elicited any additional information.

FURTHER RESEARCHES ON THE ROLE OF THE THYROID

Wagner-Jauregg continued his researches into the problem of cretinism and its treatment by embarking, together with Professor Friedrich Schlagenhaufer, on a programme of animal experiments on cretinous dogs. One of these, which he called 'Tschapperl' – a Viennese slang term which can be translated as 'silly little thing' – he kept in his apartment for more than a year. It was then sent to the Professor of Veterinary Medicine in Prague, where it remained for a year, but it was eventually returned to Wagner-Jauregg. The dogs were treated with thyroid substance which had a quick and spectacular success. The experiments proved that dogs responded to the treatment in the same way as humans.[36]

In the autumn of 1910 Wagner-Jauregg, together with Dr Diviak, began a new series of investigations. They wanted to study the beginning of cretinism at a very early age, and therefore at regular intervals they examined all children from birth in the small town where Wagner-Jauregg had centred his activities. Since there was so much cretinism there, they reckoned that there must be several cretins among the newly born in whom they could observe the development of the condition. Originally, they intended to limit the number to 100, but the interest of mothers in these investigations had been aroused to the extent that eventually 142 children, 81 boys and 61 girls, were observed. The two problems they studied were: (1) whether cretinism was inborn or acquired extrauterine, and (2) the age at which it could first be diagnosed. They concluded that symptoms appeared gradually. In some cases they disappeared spontaneously or as a result of treatment with thyroid medication. An account of these investigations was not published until 1918, some time after Diviak's death.[37]

It is strange that in all the accounts of experiments on the thyroid gland no mention was made of the role of iodine. In 1896 E. Baumann (1846–96)[38] had shown that the normal thyroid contained iodine which when given as medicine had as good results as thyroid substance in the treatment of goitre. It had long been established that endemic goitre and endemic cretinism were intimately connected and where there was no endemic goitre there was no endemic cretinism. Already in 1898, in a lecture to the Austrian Society for Health Care,[39] Wagner-Jauregg had recalled a case which demonstrated that treatment with iodine could have a beneficial effect on cretinism if the latter was associated with goitre. In 1906 he drew attention to the freedom from both goitre and cretinism in coastal areas[40] which he explained as the consequence of small amounts of iodine being atomised in the air from iodine-containing seawater. Not until his chapter on the thyroid in the *Lehrbuch der Organotherapie*,[41] which he edited together with Gustav Bayer, is the role of iodine discussed in some detail.* This chapter, as well as his contribution to G. Aschaffenburg's *Handbook of Psychiatry*, published in 1915[42], represent the final summing up of the problem that had occupied Wagner-Jauregg for more than thirty years. In them he slightly modified the thyroidal theory first put forward in 1893[43] and examined in detail in his paper of 1900.[44]

His theory had aroused a hard-fought controversy, carried on with some acrimony not only by Scholz, but especially by H. Bircher's son, E. Bircher (b. 1882), who maintained his father's belief that in cretinism no change in thyroid function had been established, and that therefore it could not be considered as the cause of the disease. In this paper of 1911[45], referring to the Scholz/Wagner-Jauregg episode, E. Bircher quoted Scholz, who had argued against Wagner-Jauregg's theory, and expressed his disbelief in the successes claimed by Wagner-Jauregg for his thyroid therapy. He concluded that cretinism was related to the thyroid only in so far as it could be caused by damage leading to struma.

Wagner-Jauregg had originally claimed that the theory that endemic cretinism was due to malfunction of the thyroid gland could account for all the symptoms of the disease, but he now admitted that it was difficult to discover the relation of imbecility and deaf-mutism to hypothyroidism. Although most symptoms of cretinism disappeared as a result of treatment with thyroid preparations, high grades of mental weakness and imbecility (and also deaf-mutism) were not cured, particularly in children more than one to two years old. The proof that imbecility and deaf mutism were entirely due to malfunction of the thyroid was therefore still lacking.

Wagner-Jauregg believed that the symptoms of sporadic and endemic cretinism were essentially the same. The success of treatment by thyroid injection or by taking thyroid extracts in cases of endemic cretinism led to the same method being applied in cases of sporadic cretinism. Again, the results as far as physical symptoms

---

*It was some years later that Wagner-Jauregg began his campaign for goitre prophylaxis by means of iodised cooking salt.

were concerned were much more satisfactory than in the case of mental defects. In one respect, however, the successes were different for the two kinds of cretinism. In sporadic cretinism, when treatment was discontinued, relapses occurred; in endemic cretinism, on the other hand, improvement continued even after treatment had ceased. This suggested that in cases of the latter there usually existed more thyroid substance capable of restitution.

The arguments relating to the nature of endemic cretinism and its symptoms and to the distinction between it and sporadic cretinism seem to have continued until fairly recently. However, at a Symposium on the subject in 1972,[46] most contributors to the Conference agreed that, although the pathogenesis of cretinism and even its relationship to the thyroid had remained obscure and controversial, it arose from insufficient thyroid hormone in foetal and neo-natal life, thus confirming Wagner-Jauregg's long held views.

REFERENCES

[1] J.L. Reverdin. Les accidents consécutifs à l'ablation totale du goitre. *Rev.Med.Suisse*, 1882, 10: 539–540; J.L. and A. Reverdin. Note sur vingt-deux operations de goitre. *Rev.Med.Suisse Romande*, 1883, 3: no. 4, 169–198; no. 5, 233–278; no. 6, 309–364.

[2] Th. Kocher. Ueber Kropfextirpationundihre Folgen. *Arch.Klin. Chir.*, 1883, 29: 254–337.

[3] Julius Wagner-Jauregg. *Lebenserinnerungen.* Ed. L. Schönbauer und M. Jantsch. Wien: Springer Verlag, 1950, p. 123.

[4] K.K. Gesellschaft der Aerzte, Wien. *Med.Jahrb.*, 1884, no. 33, 175–176.

[5] Julius Wagner-Jauregg. Ueber die Folgen der Exstirpation der Schilddrüse. *Wien.Med.Blätter*, 1884, no. 25, 771–775; no. 30, 931–935.

[6] Moritz Schiff. Bericht über eine Versuchsreihe betreffend die Wirkungen der Exstirpation der Schilddrüse. *Arch.Exp.Path.Pharmakol.*, 1884, 18: 25–34; originally publ. in *Rev.Med.Suisse Romande*, 12 Feb. 1884.

[7] Wagner-Jauregg, op.cit. ref 3, pp. 123–124.

[8] Ivar V. Sandström. On a new gland in man and several mammals. *Bull.Hist.Med.*, 1938, 6: 192–222 (transl. from *Upsala Läkaref Föch*, 1880).

[9] Wagner-Jauregg, op.cit. ref 3, pp. 125 *et seq.*

[10] Julius Wagner-Jauregg. Untersuchungen über den Cretinismus. *Jahrb.Psychiat.Neurol.*, 1893, 12: 102–137; 1894, 13: 17–36.

[11] Julius Wagner-Jauregg. Ueber den Cretinismus. *Mitteilungen des Vereins der Aerzte in Steiermark*, 1893, 30: 87–101.

[12] Kocher, op.cit. ref 2.

[13] Wagner-Jauregg, op.cit. ref 3, p. 128.

[14] Th. Kocher. Zur Verhütung des Cretinismus und cretinoider Zustände nach neuen Forschungen. *Deut.Z.Chir.*, 1892, 34: 556–626.

[15] H. Bircher. Das Myxödem und die cretinische Degeneration. *Volkmanns Sammlung klinischer Vorträge*, 1890, no. 357, 3339–3424.

[16] C.A. Ewald. *Die Erkrankungen der Schilddrüse, Myxödem und Cretinismus*. Vol. xii of H. Nothnagel. *Specielle Pathologie und Therapie*. Wien: Alfred Hölder, 1896.

[17] Wagner-Jauregg, op.cit. ref 3, p. 129.

[18] D.M. Bourneville. Notes sommaires sur deux cas d'idiotie avec *Cachexia pachydermique*. *Arch.Neurol.*, 1888, 16: 431–434.

[19] Felix Semon. A typical case of myxoedema. *Brit.Med.J.*, Dec. 1883, (ii), 1072–73.

[20] George R. Murray. The pathology of the thyroid gland. *Lancet*, 1899, (i), 667–668, 747–752.

[21] Julius Wagner-Jauregg. Ueber endemischen und sporadischen Cretinismus und dessen Behandlung. *Wien.Klin.Wschr.*, 1900, 13: no. 19, 419–427.

[22] J. Thomson. The Variation in, and the Limits of, the Improvement of Cretins at different ages under thyroid treatment. *Brit.Med.J.*, 1896, (ii), 618–620.

[23] George R. Murray. Note on the treatment of myxoedema by hypodermic injections of an extract of the thyroid gland of a sheep. *Brit.Med.J.*, 1891, (ii), 796–797.

[24] Wagner-Jauregg, op.cit. ref 3, p. 129.

[25] Ibid. p. 130.

[26] Wilhelm Scholz. Zur Lehre vom Cretinismus. *Wien.Klin.Wschr.*, 1902, 15: no. 22, 592–593.

[27] Julius Wagner-Jauregg. Zur Behandlung des endemischen Cretinismus. *Wien.Klin.Wschr.*, 1902, 15: no. 25, 651–652.

[28] Wagner-Jauregg, op.cit. ref 3, p. 134.

[29] Julius Wagner-Jauregg. Beitrag zur Behandlung des endemischen Cretinismus. *Mitteilungen des Vereins der Aerzte in Steiermark*, 1903, 40: 271–275.

[30] Wagner-Jauregg, op.cit. ref 3, p. 134.

[31] Ibid. p. 135; and *Verhandlungen des Kongresses für Innere Medizin*, 23. Kongress, München, April 1906. Wiesbaden: 1906.

[32] Julius Wagner-Jauregg. Ueber Behandlung des endemischen Kretinismus mit Schilddrüsensubstanz. *Wien.Klin.Wschr.*, 1904, 17: no. 30, 835–841; 1907, 20: no. 2, 33–42.

[33] Wagner-Jauregg, op.cit. ref 3, pp. 135–136.

[34] Manuscript held at Institut für Geschichte der Medizin der Universität Wien.

[35] F. Hochstetter. Julius Wagner-Jauregg. *Akademie der Wissenschaften in Wien, Almanach* für das Jahr 1941, 91: 197–203; O. Pötzl. *Wien.Klin.Wschr.*, 1940, 53: 4 p.

[36] Julius Wagner-Jauregg und Friedrich Schlagenhaufer. *Beiträge zur Aetiologie und Pathologie des endemischen Kretinismus*. Wien/Leipzig: F. Deuticke, 1910.

[37] Roman Diviak und Julius Wagner-Jauregg. Ueber die Entstehung des endemischen Kretinismus in den ersten Lebensjahren. *Wien.Klin.Wschr.*, 1918, 31: no. 6, 149–162.

[38] E. Baumann. Ueber den Jodgehalt der Schilddrüsen von Menschen und Tieren. *Z.Physiol.Chem.*, 1896, 22: 1–17.

[39] Julius Wagner-Jauregg. Ueber den Kretinismus. *Monatsschr. Gesundheitspflege*. 1898, 16: no. 3, 57–68.

[40] Julius Wagner-Jauregg. Ueber marinen Kretinismus. *Wien.Klin.Wschr.*, 1906, 29: no. 43, 1273–78.

[41] Julius Wagner-Jauregg. 'Schilddrüse'. In: *Lehrbuch der Organotherapie*, hrsg. Wagner v. Jauregg und Gustav Bayer. Leipzig: Georg Thieme, 1914, pp. 88–154.

[42] Julius Wagner-Jauregg. 'Myxoedem und Kretinismus'. In: *Handbuch der Psychiatrie*, hrsg. G. Aschaffenburg. Leipzig/Wien: F. Deuticke, 1915, Spezieller Teil, 2. Abteilung, 1. Hälfte.

[43] Wagner-Jauregg, op.cit. ref 11.

[44] Wagner-Jauregg, op.cit. ref 21.

[45] E. Bircher. 'Fortfall und Aenderung der Schilddrüsenfunktion als Krankheitsursachen'. In: O. Lubarsch und R. Ostertag, hrsg. *Ergebnisse der allgemeinen Pathologie und pathologischen Anatomie des Menschen und der Tiere*, 1911, 15: 1 Abt., 82–377.

[46] B.S. Hetzel. In: J.B. Stanbury and R.L. Kroc, Ed. *Human development and the thyroid gland. Relation to endemic cretinism*. Proceedings of a Symposium on Endemic Cretinism held at the Kroc Foundation, Santa Ynez Valley, California, 24–26 Jan. 1972. (*Advances in Experimental Medicine and Biology*, 30) New York/London: Plenum Press, pp. 119–134.

NINE

THE CAMPAIGN FOR GOITRE PREVENTION THROUGH IODISED SALT

In his *Memoirs* Wagner-Jauregg wrote that, with the publication, together with Dr Diviak, of his investigations of cretinism among children in the small town in Styria where he had centred his activities, his work on the problem of the thyroid had been completed. However, when at the end of the First World War the incidence of goitre, particularly in the mountainous regions of Austria, had assumed alarming proportions, he was once again led to resume work on a subject that was intimately connected with the problem of the thyroid, that of goitre. He was fully aware that endemic cretinism and endemic goitre were connected, and that where there was no endemic goitre there was no endemic cretinism. At one time, the fact that not all cretins suffered from goitre had raised some doubt as to the relation of goitre and cretinism, but it was found that goitre-free cretins suffered from an atrophied thyroid and that atrophy or goitrous thyroid both led to the mal-function of the gland.

The first to establish that iodine was necessary for thyroid function were D. Marine (1880–1976) and O.P. Kimball,[1] who were led to experiment on pigs and sheep, suffering from goitrous degeneration of the thyroid, by treating them with iodine. Their iodine prophylaxis worked so well that they later tried it on humans with equal success. Actually, the first to prescribe iodine in the treatment of goitre was J.F. Coindet (1774–1834) in 1833, nearly a hundred years earlier.[2] He was followed in 1854 by G.A. Chatin (1813–1901),[3] who recommended that the water supply in goitrous districts should be supplemented with iodine. His work fell into discredit and oblivion until it was resuscitated nearly seventy years later. The first to suggest the iodization of salt for the prevention of goitre was J.B. Boussingault (1801–87) in 1833.[4] In Austria it was F. Koestl in 1855 who proposed the use of iodised salt.[5]

As recounted in the previous chapter on cretinism, Wagner-Jauregg had already in 1898, in a lecture to the Austrian Society for Health Care, proposed the use of iodine in the treatment of cretinism.[6] He suggested that in areas where goitre and cretinism were endemic very small amounts of sodium iodide should be added to cooking salt, which could be done easily in Austria where there was a salt State monopoly. In view of Wagner-Jauregg's interest in the problem, it is not surprising that, at the end of the First World War, the Austrian Office of Public Health, alarmed by the increase in the incidence of goitre, asked him to give his expert opinion on an article by R. Klinger on 'The prevention of endemic goitre', published in one of the weekly medical periodicals.[7] In his report[8] Wagner-Jauregg referred to his 1898 lecture which was in agreement with Klinger's proposals. Klinger claimed that only large scale attempts for the supply of iodine were likely to bring progress in the prevention of goitre. He himself once a week gave pupils in country schools in areas where goitre was endemic a tablet containing cocoa and sugar and also either 2–3 mg of sodium iodide or 10–20 mg of iodised stearinic acid corresponding to 5–10 mg of iodine. Other Swiss workers had made similar experiments with surprisingly favourable results.

However, Wagner-Jauregg thought that methods like Klinger's were not suitable for the large-scale and continuous application which was necessary if the whole population of a goitrous area was to become free from goitre and cretinism. These methods were cumbersome and could only be applied in schools, whereas it was important to treat children from birth and to continue treatment after school age. The method of adding iodine to cooking salt had the advantage of acting on the whole population, without exception, from the moment of conception. Moreover, it did not depend on the conscientiousness of individual people and could not be undermined by the indolence of one particular person.

Klinger, like Wagner-Jauregg believed in principle that iodine should be added to cooking salt, but he thought that a general issue of iodine tablets to school children should precede its introduction, since he feared that hypersensitive people could suffer damage as a result and develop hyperthyroidism and Basedow.* Wagner-Jauregg denied that the small amounts of iodine added could have these damaging effects. Although he admitted that cases of Basedow could occur through the medicinal use of iodine salts, he argued that in these cases the daily amount ingested must have been at least decigrams, not milligrams. The small amounts envisaged for addition to cooking salt were more likely to be similar to those many people took daily in their diet, and they could do no damage. He even claimed that small amounts of iodine salts could be beneficial in the treatment of Basedow's disease.

Iodised cooking salt introduced in Austria

Wagner-Jauregg therefore advised the Office of Public Health to adopt his proposal, made as early as 1898, to introduce into areas of endemic goitre cooking salt containing 2 mg per kilo of iodine salts (either potassium or sodium iodide) and to abandon experiments with iodine-containing tablets. To control the effect of this measure it would be necessary to count the number of goitres before and during its application in a few schools.

In two lectures in 1923, one to the Vienna Medical Society[9] and the other given in conjunction with the 10th International Course on Further Education organised by the Vienna Medical School[10], Wagner-Jauregg spoke at greater length on the aetiology, therapy and prevention of goitre. In these he referred to the excellent results obtained by Swiss physicians, particularly O. Bayard (1812–52): in all the persons treated with iodine goitre had disappeared. Wagner-Jauregg showed pictures of four children in all of whom goitre had vanished.

In considering the financial problems of producing iodised salt, Wagner-Jauregg thought that by increasing the price of all cooking salt by a small amount in goitrous areas the extra cost would be covered. As far as problems of manufacture were concerned, mostly in connection with the even distribution of the iodine in the salt, the Swiss had developed a satisfactory method.[11]

Following Wagner-Jauregg's advice to the Office of Public Health, the principal of the Department took an interest in the proposal, and a meeting was held during the summer of 1922 at

---

* Exophthalmic goitre.

which the method of producing iodised salt was discussed. As a result iodised cooking salt with a 5 mg content per kilo was introduced in Austria in the autumn of 1923. It was produced in the state saltmines and distributed so that it could be bought wherever it was asked for. However, the ultimate aim of the project was to sell the iodised salt in all areas where goitre was endemic and only to issue the uniodised salt on request.[12] Wagner-Jauregg appealed to colleagues with practices in goitrous districts (and in Austria that meant a great part of the country) to make propaganda for the iodised salt, to recommend it not only to those families where one or more members were afflicted, but to everybody to prevent goitre. An essential part of the campaign was that the price was to be the same as for ordinary salt.

OPPOSITION TO GOITRE PROPHYLAXIS

Because Wagner-Jauregg had been responsible for the introduction of iodised salt in Austria, he felt it incumbent on him to report on the results, to examine objections from medical quarters and to consider whether they were justified.[13] Claims had been made that since then the incidence of hyperthyroid disease had greatly increased both in Austria and in Switzerland. The publicity following the introduction of iodised salt had led people suffering from goitre to procure iodine which was available without medical prescription. Moreover, pharmaceutical companies had begun to produce and advertise iodine preparations, mostly in tablet form and often in dangerously high doses. Thus, many persons suffering from goitre had been taking iodine without medical advice and consequently had developed symptoms of Basedow's disease. Wagner-Jauregg urged that, to avoid this happening, medicines containing iodine should be made available only on medical prescription.

From Austrian medical quarters criticism came first from J. Wiesel (b. 1876),[14] who claimed that damage could result from iodised cooking salt. He based his claim on statements by E. Bircher[15] that, as a result of the introduction of iodised cooking salt, there had been an increase of cases of Basedow and many cases of iodine damage. These were, however, contradicted by the results of an enquiry of all Swiss general practitioners, organised by the Swiss Office of Health at the end of 1924 at the suggestion of the Swiss Goitre Commission. Its purpose was to determine the incidence of Basedow and the degree of possible damage, following the introduction of goitre prophylaxis through iodised cooking salt. It was found that only very few cases of hyperthyroidism were due to the use of iodised salt, and the Swiss Office of Health issued a report to this effect to the daily press. (A critical assessment of the results was published by W. Flück some four years later.[16] In his view the advantages of the use of iodised salt far outweighed the disadvantages.) Nevertheless, Bircher remained adamant that iodised salt was dangerous. Wagner-Jauregg therefore got in touch with a number of Swiss physicians who were advocating goitre prophylaxis, including F. de Quervain (1868–1940), H. Eggenberger (1881–1946) and H. Hunziker (1878–1941), to find out more details of the results of the enquiry. They all confirmed his views and he therefore advised the Austrian Office of Public Health to follow the example of the Swiss and not to believe claims of damage through iodised cooking salt without checking their correctness.

Already before the introduction of iodised cooking salt, opponents of the project had argued that there were people who could suffer as a result of the minute doses of iodine in iodised salt. Wagner-Jauregg was certain that without iodine the thyroid could not function. Investigations carried out by Fellenberg[17] showed that in goitre-free areas the daily content of iodine passed in urine was 64γ (1γ = one millionth part of a gram), whereas in goitrous regions it was only about 18γ. The daily intake by using iodised salt was 40γ, and thus well within the physiological amount of daily iodine metabolism. If these small doses of iodine were damaging, then persons moving from iodine-poor regions to iodine-rich areas would be adversely affected, which was not the case. Fellenberg claimed that a person drinking one pint of milk and eating a few eggs from a goitre-free area would have taken more iodine than was contained in a daily dose of iodised salt.

The results of experiments by Kaspar,[18] who had treated a great number of goitrous persons with very small doses of iodine (40γ), showed a startling diminution in the number of goitres. In 300 to 400 cases there was only one single patient on whom the dose used in cooking salt had an adverse effect.

In 1927 an International Goitre Conference was held in Berne[19] at which the problem of goitre-prevention by the introduction of iodised salt was discussed. In an opening speech E. Bircher claimed that, although iodine played an important role in goitre, other factors were equally significant. In his view, absence of iodine as a cause of goitre could not be proved. False hopes had been raised of iodine prophylaxis and therapy. However, most of those attending the Conference spoke in favour of the fight against goitre by means of iodine, and arguments that iodised salt could have a damaging effect were dismissed. A distinction was made between endemic goitre, or alpine goitre, and the type of goitre, usually called Danzig goitre, which is found in plains and coastal regions. The latter is never associated with cretinism and is sensitive to iodine. If malfunction of the thyroid is involved, it is mostly a case of hyperthyroidism and not of hypothyroidism as in alpine goitre. The aetiology of goitre was discussed at some length and, although various theories were put forward, it was generally agreed that endemic goitre occurred where the provision of iodine was insufficient. Wagner-Jauregg, who was present at the Conference, argued[20] that damaging effects as a result of iodised cooking salt were most unlikely, since through its intake the organism only absorbed 0.02 to 0.03 mg of iodine daily, iodine secretion amounting to 0.03 to 0.94 mg. The minimum daily amount of iodine that could lead to hyperthyroidism was 0.5 to 1.0 mg, a higher dose. However, it was almost impossible to prove in individual cases the causal relationship between damage and the use of iodised salt, because many medicaments containing large doses of iodine were dispensed without indication of their iodine content. Wagner-Jauregg believed, as did the Swiss School, in the close relation of cretinism and goitre to thyroid disease. He was sceptical of the assumption that an infection or emanation of radium through soil or water could cause goitre.

RESULTS OF GOITRE PROPHYLAXIS

In 1928, although it was still too early to assess fully the results of the introduction of iodised cooking salt in Austria (this could not be possible until the children who had been fed on it had become of school age), some data became available which indicated the beneficial effect of iodised salt. In Vienna, according to statistics prepared by the City Health Office, the incidence of goitre, particularly severe goitre, showed a definite decrease in primary and secondary schools between 1923 and 1927.[21] The figures show that in elementary schools goitre formation had fallen from 42.1 per cent to 31.7 per cent, i.e. by about 10 per cent, and in high schools from 47.8 per cent to 43.2 per cent, i.e. about 5 per cent. The degree of improvement was even more marked in cases of severe goitres. However, it was difficult to decide whether this was due to iodised cooking salt (which in Vienna represented 47 per cent of salt sold) or whether the increase in goitre after the war had abated.

Results for school children in some Austrian provinces for the same years (1923 and 1927) also showed a distinct decrease in the incidence of goitre, particularly in the Tirol, a mountainous region. Some even more significant statistics were collected for the years 1923, 1931 and 1936 in a district of Styria where iodised cooking salt was introduced for the whole population. There the number of goitres had fallen, in the case of boys, from 62.33 per cent in 1923 to 53.9 per cent in 1931 and to 36.5 per cent in 1936, and, in the case of girls, from 67.42 per cent to 56.6 per cent and 41.48 per cent, respectively. The decrease was particularly marked in the younger age groups who had been eating iodised cooking salt longest.[22]

Wagner-Jauregg also made an enquiry of all surgical clinics in Vienna and Lower Austria and found that since the introduction of iodised salt the number of operations of goitre had fallen by 40 per cent in Vienna and about 20 per cent in Lower Austria. Although he thought that this might be partly due to goitre sufferers having been made aware of the iodine treatment and postponing the operation, he believed that urgent goitre operations could not be put off indefinitely.[23]

THE CAMPAIGN AGAINST IODISED COOKING SALT

In Switzerland the use of iodised cooking salt varied from canton to canton: in some it was in general use, whereas in others it was not. In view of this, the supporters of goitre prophylaxis demanded that the introduction of iodised salt should be made obligatory for the whole of the country.[24] As a result, the Swiss Goitre Commission proposed to the Government that this should be done. The leader of the campaign against the use of iodised cooking salt, E. Bircher, vehemently opposed this step.[25] He claimed that the general distribution of iodine threatened the health of the people. He published a list of authors, including many Americans, who had voiced their opposition to iodised cooking salt. In reply, F. de Quervain argued[26] that Bircher had failed to point out that the iodised salt used in America contained about forty times the amount of iodine present in the Swiss salt. He pleaded for goitre prevention. 'Doctors,' he wrote, 'should no longer be blamed that they can only operate on goitre, but not prevent it.'

Nevertheless, in the early 1930s the campaign against iodised salt gathered momentum. Once again in February 1931 a general enquiry was organised by the Swiss Medical Weekly, of which Bircher was one of the editors.[27] A questionnaire was sent to authors in Switzerland and abroad. One of the questions was 'Do you consider the uncontrolled distribution of iodine preparations or iodine cooking salt damaging or dangerous?' This was clearly an unfair question since the effect of iodised cooking salt differed greatly from that of iodine preparations in general and the question ought to have been in two parts. Wagner-Jauregg[28] thought that the question was badly worded and the answers poorly analysed, since it was iodised cooking salt that was in question, not other iodine preparations. He himself believed that damage due to iodised salt was most unlikely. It seemed nonsensical to him to maintain that minimum amounts of iodine could have any adverse effect, since we absorb and secrete iodine daily.

In Austria F. Högler and W. Raab were the most vociferous opponents of Wagner-Jauregg's efforts towards the general introduction of iodised cooking salt. Högler[29] in two papers on the treatment of hypothyroidism denied the beneficial effect of iodised cooking salt, which he believed could lead to hyperthyroidism. He claimed that the majority of cases were due to it and he thought that it should be banned. The poorer members of the community were in the greater danger because they ate far more cooked meats, sausages and bread, in the preparation of which much salt was used.

The other opponent of goitre prophylaxis through iodised cooking salt, W. Raab,[30] in his articles quoted many cases of damage due to iodine medication among the Viennese population. He thought that Fellenberg's arguments that the daily intake of iodine by using iodised cooking salt was well within the physiological amount of daily iodine metabolism were fallacious, because biological iodine was different from potassium iodide in salt. When he presented one of these papers to a meeting of the Vienna Medical Society[31] several speakers, including Wagner-Jauregg and de Quervain, argued that the deleterious effects of iodine observed were not due to iodised cooking salt, but to the uncontrolled use of medicines containing iodine, such as mouth washes, ointments and suppositories. It was untrue, de Quervain claimed, that iodised cooking salt was used in the preparation of meat products, sausages and bread, as claimed by Högler.

In the campaign for and against goitre prophylaxis by means

of iodised cooking salt, which in Austria began in 1922 (some time later than in Switzerland), the arguments were largely based on case histories on the one side and statistics on the other. The opponents of the campaign blamed the incidence of hyperthyroidism on the intake of iodine through iodised cooking salt, where as those in favour tried to show that it had usually been caused by intake of iodine in some other form. Iodine in fairly large doses appeared in all kinds of disguises and many iodine-containing preparations were available for sale without medical prescription. Their name often did not suggest that they contained iodine and sometimes even physicians were ignorant of that fact. Wagner-Jauregg[32] questioned the diagnosis of hyperthyroidism in some of the cases. This had become a common-place description to conceal the failure to make a correct diagnosis of some functional nervous disorders. Moreover, the possibility of the patient having taken iodine in far larger doses than were present in iodised cooking salt, sometimes even without his knowledge, was considerable.

Wagner-Jauregg accused his opponents of bringing pressure to bear on the Salt Mines Office by claiming that the medical profession was against the distribution of iodised salt and by insinuating that it might have to deal with claims for damages by those who had suffered adverse effects by its use. Thus the Office ordered that as from 1 January 1933, iodised cooking salt would no longer be sold in sacks, but only in packets of one kilo at a much higher price. This, according to Wagner-Jauregg, undermined the hope of goitre prophylaxis through iodised cooking salt because an essential assumption making its widespread introduction possible was that its cost was no higher than that of non-iodised salt. Wagner-Jauregg, in pessimistic mood, concluded that this was effectively the end of goitre prophylaxis. To adopt Raab's proposal to carry it out in individual cases only with medical supervision would be utterly foolish and pervert the essential purpose of the campaign.

THE AETIOLOGY OF GOITRE

Throughout the campaign questions of the aetiology of goitre seemed to have been raised only incidentally. Although the 1927 Conference decided that iodine was effective as a means of prevention, it was not unanimous on the theory of iodine deficiency as the sole cause of goitre. Bayard in 1923 had called endemic goitre a deficiency disease,[33] but Bircher in 1927 claimed that absence of iodine as a cause of goitre could not be proved.[34] Wagner-Jauregg in a paper in 1932,[35] dealt with the aetiology of goitre at some length in the light of current literature. Speaking of the theory that lack of iodine was the cause of goitre, he referred to the small difference in the amount of iodine available to those with and without goitre. In his opinion, it was not this which differentiated them but the inability of those with goitre to maintain the normal function of the thyroid without increasing its size. The fault did not lie with the amount of iodine, but with the thyroid and it was therefore necessary to assume some damage to the thyroid by an unknown cause. Conditions which encouraged or prevented the occurrence of endemic goitre, such as the nature of the soil on the one hand and plenty of iodine provision on the other were known, but the cause of the appearance of goitre in so many parts of the globe was not. A recent work on the subject[36] refers to the arguments of some observers who were unwilling to accept an aetiological relationship between iodine deficiency on the one hand and goitre and cretinism on the other. It does, however, conclude that the strongest argument for iodine deficiency as the most important aetiological factor in goitre and cretinism is that wherever iodine prophylaxis has been put into effect, there has been a spectacular disappearance of endemic cretinism.

THE FATE OF GOITRE PROPHYLAXIS

Although in his article of 1933[37] Wagner-Jauregg spoke of the end of goitre prophylaxis as a result of the price increase in iodised cooking salt as compared with the non-iodised, he persevered in his fight for it. In Austria he was the lonely upholder of the campaign, whereas in Switzerland the vociferous opponent E. Bircher had a number of fighters against him. In several cantons iodised cooking salt was available, but according to Merke[38] its success was limited because it was not being used widely enough and contained too little iodine. However, the statistics he quoted showed that there was no doubt about the beneficial effect of iodised cooking salt. During the last few years of his life when Wagner-Jauregg was already a very sick man he continued to write on the subject. In two articles he reviewed the progress of goitre prophylaxis in different countries and pleaded for more statistics to show its success.[39] He was aware that goitre prophylaxis had to be aimed at children and that it had to begin during pregnancy. The only way to reach all mothers was through iodised cooking salt and therefore individual treatment of goitre would defeat the object of the campaign.

In a book published two years before his death he wrote an account of the fight against goitre and of goitre prophylaxis in Austria.[40] In a short review in the Swiss Medical Weekly, Bircher, his long-standing opponent, although he said that he was not justified in voicing his criticism because he was against Wagner-Jauregg's theory, nevertheless went on to criticise Wagner-Jauregg's claims that goitre and cretinism had diminished. However, the Third Goitre Conference held in Washington in 1938, on which Wagner-Jauregg wrote a report[41] based on the Official Report, agreed that there was no reason to think that iodine in the small amounts which prevented goitre had any deleterious effects.

In his own country, Wagner-Jauregg lived to see the end of goitre prophylaxis as a result of an order by the Ministry of the Interior issued in November 1938, warning against the use of iodine-containing drugs and iodised salt. This marked the end of goitre prophylaxis through iodised cooking salt in Austria for some years. Alas, Wagner-Jauregg died before the order was rescinded in October 1944, as a result of the frightening increase in the occurrence of goitre, and iodised cooking salt became readily available again. Thus, Wagner-Jauregg's campaign, which occupied so much of his time and energy during the last twenty years of his life, eventually succeeded and his heroic efforts to improve the health of the nation were found not to have been in vain.

Not until 1963 was a new law regarding the iodization of salt adopted by the National Assembly of Austria. According to this, edible salt described as 'Vollsalz' (full salt) may only be offered for sale if it contains 10 mg of potassium iodide per kilogram. Non-iodized salt must be marked accordingly and not sold as 'full salt'; moreover, it must only be sold at the express wish of the buyer. The law was amended in 1990 raising the addition of potassium iodide to 20 mg per kilogram. It is ironical that the addition of 2 mg of iodine salt per kilogram of cooking salt, originally proposed by Wagner-Jauregg and opposed by so many of his contemporaries, has now been increased ten times.

REFERENCES

[1] D. Marine and O.P. Kimball. The prevention of simple goitre in man. *J.Labor.Clin.Med.*, 1917, 3: 40; *Arch.Int.Med.*, 1918, 23: 41;

Am.J.Med.Sci., 1922, 163: 634; *J.Am.Med.Assoc.*, 1919, p. 1873.

2 Jean Francois Coindet. Découverte d'un nouveau remède contre le goitre. *Ann.Chim.Phys.*, 1820, 14: 190–198; 15: 45–59.

3 G.A. Chatin. Recherche de l'iode dans l'air, les eaux, le sol et les produits alimentaires des Alpes de la France et du Piemont. *Compt.Rend.Acad.Sci.Paris*, 1852, 34: 14–18; Recherche comparative de l'iode et de quelques autres principes dans les eaux (et les egouts) qui alimentent Paris, Londres et Turin. Ibid. 35: 127–130; Recherche de l'iode dans l'air, les eaux, le sol et les produits alimentaires du Jura, du Valais, de la Lombardie, de l'Allemagne et de la Belgique. Ibid. 1854, 38: 83–85.

4 J.B. Boussingault. Sur l'existence de l'iode dans l'eau d'une saline de la province d'Antioquia. *Ann.Chim.Phys.*, 1825, vol. 40; 1831, vol. 48; 1833, 54: 163.

5 F. Koestl. *Der endemische Kretinismus als Gegenstand der öffentlichen Fürsorge.* Wien: 1855.

6 Julius Wagner-Jauregg. Ueber den Kretinismus. *Monatsschr. Gesundheitspflege*, 1898, 16: no. 3.

7 R. Klinger. Die Kropfprophylaxe des endemischen Kropfes. *Wien.Klin.Wschr.*, 1922, 35: no. 2, 35–37.

8 Julius Wagner-Jauregg. Die Behandlung und Prophylaxe des endemischen Kropfes. *Wien.Klin.Wschr.*, 1922, 35: no. 16, 369–370.

9 Julius Wagner-Jauregg. Zur Therapie und Prophylaxe des Kropfes. *Wien.Klin.Wschr.*, 1923, 36: no. 8, 139–142.

10 Julius Wagner-Jauregg. Vorbeugung des Kropfes. *Wien.Med. Wschr.*, 1923, 73: no. 47, 2090–96.

11 Op.cit. ref 9.

12 Op.cit. ref 10.

13 Julius Wagner-Jauregg. Kropfprophylaxe durch Vollsalz. *Wien. Klin.Wschr.*, 1925, 38: no. 48, 1377–80.

14 J. Wiesel. Ueber Zunahme des M. Basedow und von Thyreosen in Wien nebst Bemerkungen über die Jodtherapie obiger Syndrome. *Med.Klinik*, 1925, 21: no. 39, 1445–48.

15 E. Bircher. Zur Jodbehandlung des Kropfes. *Klin.Wschr.*, 1925, 4: no. 16, 742–745.

16 W. Flück. Die schweizerische Basedowstatistik von 1922–24. Ein Beitrag zur Kenntnis des Jodbasedow. *Schweiz.Med.Wschr.*, 1928, 9: no. 1, 2–12; no. 2, 28–36.

17 T. von Fellenberg. *Mitt.Lebensmitt.*, 1923, 24: 123.

18 F. Kaspar. Jodschäden durch 'kleine' Jodgaben und ihre Vermeidung. *Wien.Med.Wschr.*, 1924, 74: no. 34, 1758–59; Individuelle

Jodminimumtherapie und Rezidivstruma. *Wien.Klin.Wschr.*, 1924, 37: no. 28, 705–706.

[19] Der internationalen Kropfkonferenz in Bern 24.–25.Aug. 1927 gewidmet. *Schweiz.Med.Wschr.*, 1927, 8: no. 34, 801–828; no. 35, 829–854.

[20] Julius Wagner-Jauregg. Endemischer Kropf und Myxoedem. *Wien.Klin.Wschr.*, 1930, 43: no. 1, 1–6.

[21] Julius Wagner-Jauregg. Vorläufiger Bericht über Erfolge der Kropfprophylaxe. *Wien.Klin.Wschr.*, 1928, 41: no. 24, 833–836.

[22] Julius Wagner-Jauregg. Der Kampf um das Vollsalz. *Wien.Klin. Wschr.*, 1934, 47: no. 11, 321–323; Ueber die Ausbreitung der Kropfprophylaxe durch jodiertes Speisesalz. *Wien.Klin.Wschr.*, 1937, 50: no. 20, 797–799.

[23] Wagner-Jauregg, op.cit. ref 21.

[24] O. Stiner. Jodiertes Kochsalz für die ganze Schweiz. *Schweiz.Med. Wschr.*, 1928, 9: no. 41, 1014–16.

[25] E. Bircher. Jodiertes Kochsalz für die ganze Schweiz. *Schweiz. Med.Wschr.*, 1919, 10: no. 6, 123–126.

[26] F. de Quervain. Zur Kropfprophylaxe durch jodiertes Kochsalz. *Schweiz.Med.Wschr.*, 1929, 10: no. 44, 1099–1101.

[27] Kropfumfrage. *Schweiz.Med.Wschr.*, 1932, 13: no. 25, 582–587; no. 26, 607–610.

[28] Julius Wagner-Jauregg. Das Ende der Kropfprophylaxe durch Vollsalz. *Wien.Klin.Wschr.*, 1933, 46: no. 1, 5–9.

[29] F. Högler. Ueber die Radiumbehandlung des Morbus Basedowii und der Hyperthyreosen. *Wien.Klin.Wschr.*, 1931, 44: no. 6, 180–184; Therapie der Hyperthyreosen vom internen Standpunkte. Ibid. no. 31, 1002–1003; *Wien.Med.Wschr.*, 1932, 82: no. 36, 1135–40.

[30] W. Raab. Jodschäden in der Wiener Bevölkerung. *Wien.Klin. Wschr.*, 1931, 44: no. 8, 273–276; no. 10, 309–317; Zur Frage der Jodempfindlichkeit Erwachsener. *Wien.Med.Wschr.*, 1932, 82: no. 50, 1549–52.

[31] Raab, op.cit. *Wien.Klin.Wschr.*, ref 30.

[32] Julius Wagner-Jauregg. Die angeblichen Schilddrüsenschädigungen durch Vollsalz. *Wien.Klin.Wschr.*, 1931, 44: no. 10, 317–320; 1933, 46: no. 1, 5–9.

[33] O. Bayard. *Beiträge zur Schilddrüsenfrage.* Basel: 1919; *Schweiz.Med. Wschr.*, 1923, 53: no. 30, 703–707; no. 31, 732–737.

[34] E. Bircher. Die Kropffrage. *Schweiz.Med.Wschr.*, 1927, 57: no. 34, 801.

[35] Julius Wagner-Jauregg. Ueber Kropfaetiologie. *Wien.Med.Wschr.*,

1932, 82: no. 43, 1339–43; no. 44, 1367–71.

[36] J.H. Means, L.J. deGroot and J.B. Stanbury. *The thyroid and its diseases*. 5th ed. New York: John Wiley and Sons, 1984. p. 657.

[37] Wagner-Jauregg, op.cit. ref 28.

[38] F. Merke. Die hundertjährige Leidensgeschichte der Jodprophylaxe des endemischen Kropfes. *Gesnerus*, 1974, 31: 47–53.

[39] Julius Wagner-Jauregg. Der Kampf um das Vollsalz. *Wien.Klin. Wschr.*, 1934, 47: no. 11, 321–323; Ueber die Ausbreitung der Kropfprophylaxe durch jodiertes Speisesalz. *Wien.Klin.Wschr.*, 1937, 50: no. 20, 797–799.

[40] Julius Wagner-Jauregg. *Kropfbekämpfung und Kropfverhütung in Oesterreich*. Wien: Springer Verlag, 1938; reviewed by E. Bircher. *Schweiz.Med.Wschr.*, 1938, 68: 1388.

[41] Julius Wagner-Jauregg. Einige Ergebnisse der in Washington 1938 abgehaltenen 3. Internationalen Kropfkonferenz. *Wien.Med.Wschr.*, 1939, 89: no. 45, 1057–58.

TEN

Wagner-Jauregg and Fever Therapy

T he idea that fever can have a curative effect on mental diseases goes back to antiquity. Hippocrates mentioned the
beneficial influence of a malaria infection on epilepsy and
Galen cited a case of melancholy cured as a result of an attack of
quartan fever.[1] Sydenham and Boerhaave knew of the beneficial
effect of feverish illnesses on madness. Many other instances of a
cure or remission of a mental illness as the result of a feverish illness
have been quoted in the literature, particularly during the second
half of the nineteenth century.

It was not this literature that aroused Julius Wagner-Jauregg's
interest at first, but a series of observations at the Asylum of Lower
Austria in Vienna, soon after he began work there. On 28 January
1883 a woman patient contracted an attack of erysipelas and subsequently recovered from a severe mental illness. Anxious to ascertain whether the relationship between psychoses and fever was causal
or purely incidental, he began a thorough search of the literature, as
a result of which he wrote a lengthy article on 'The effect of feverish
diseases on psychoses', published in 1887.[2] In this he reviewed
previous articles on the subject, and also related cases from his
own experience. By this time he had gained considerable clinical
experience.

In the literature he found many observations on the effects of
typhoid, cholera, intermittent fevers, acute exanthemata and erysipelas on psychoses. Most reported instances involved typhoid, because
typhoid epidemics often occurred in lunatic asylums and their effects
had been documented by several observers. Some mental patients
were cured and others temporarily improved after an attack of

typhoid. Wagner-Jauregg himself had observed a case of a woman admitted to his Clinic suffering from acute insanity, who several months later was taken ill with typhoid. She became quite normal for a short period, but eventually reverted to the severe insanity for which she had originally been admitted.[3] In another case a patient of Wagner-Jauregg suffering from epilepsy was completely cured of this, though not entirely of his insanity, after a serious attack of intermittent fever.[4] There were also reports of the beneficial effect of smallpox, including complete cures of patients suffering from general paralysis of the insane (GPI). Erysipelas, too, was reported to have had a curative effect on insane patients. Wagner-Jauregg described two cases in his paper of 1887.[5] One patient was complately cured; in the other the cure was only temporary, although her condition after the infection was not as bad as it had been before. A third patient, whose case was reported to Wagner-Jauregg by a colleague, completely recovered from severe paranoia after an attack of erysipelas. There are many references in the literature to cures of GPI following attacks of anthrax and inflammation and suppuration caused by different agents. Wagner-Jauregg mentioned three of these specifically.[6]

All the cases reported left Wagner-Jauregg in no doubt that infectious diseases could lead to the cure of mentally ill patients. The manner in which these cures were effected varied greatly. In some cases the improvement lasted only while the patient was affected by the somatic illness; in others it continued for weeks or months; in many the symptoms of insanity disappeared with the onset of the fever, in others after the patient had recovered from it. Speculating on the mechanism of these cures, Wagner-Jauregg compared the problem to that of solving an equation with two unknown quantities: neither the changes occurring in psychoses nor the ways in which feverish illnesses acted on the nervous system were known. Any attempt at an explanation had to take into account the fact that the same agent that in one case cured a disease could produce it in another, since psychoses can be brought about by certain feverish diseases. Feverish illnesses had a beneficial effect not only on psychoses, they could also favourably affect somatic diseases, erysipelas and acute exanthemata being particularly effective in this respect. For example, acute exanthemata could result in the disappearance of some chronic skin diseases. Their action was assumed to strengthen the organism.

The fact that feverish conditions only sometimes resulted

in cures led Wagner-Jauregg to enquire about the favourable circumstances. He tabulated the cases by sex and age, and by whether there was a complete cure, a significant lasting improvement, a temporary improvement, or no improvement at all.[7] His tables were based on 95 cases of typhoid, seven of typhus, three of cholera, ten of intermittent fever, twenty-two of recurrent fever, fifteen of acute exanthemata and eleven of erysipelas, the last being the most effective.

FEVER THERAPY

As a result of his researches, Wagner-Jauregg began to speculate whether it would be justifiable to generate fever as a therapy for psychoses. In this connection, he had in mind the vaccination experiments by Köstl and Kiernan;[8] the use of blood transfusions by Leidesdorf[9]; and injections of recurrent fever by A.S. Rosenblum (reported by B. Oks and J. Motschukoffsky).[10] He felt that, although the evidence was then insufficient, it did justify continuing research. It would also be necessary, he thought, to collect statistics of the effect of infections occurring naturally with mental patients. Those diseases that harmed the patient and could not be controlled and those that could not be produced artificially had to be excluded from therapeutic use: that left intermittent fevers and erysipelas. Both could be produced artificially; the former could be treated with quinine and the latter was considered a benign disease. Summarizing his studies, Wagner-Jauregg concluded that psychoses could be cured by fever. Consequently, it was necessary to study the conditions under which a cure took place.

Eight years elapsed before Wagner-Jauregg again wrote on the subject. His duties at the Psychiatric Clinic were arduous, particularly after its Director, Professor Leidesdorf, suffered a heart attack and Wagner-Jauregg had to take over both the Clinic's administration and Leidesdorf's lectures. Nevertheless, he pursued his researches, both experimental and theoretical, despite the inadequacy of the facilities at his disposal, and he continued his observations. During the winter of 1888/89 he inoculated several patients with a culture of streptococci originating from erysipelas,[11] with negative results.[12] After this disappointment he temporarily abandoned his experiments and only resumed them in 1890.

In a lecture to the Vienna Medical Society in February 1895[13] on efforts to cure insanity he recalled Professor L. Mauthner's (1840–94) report of a case of a long-standing progressive atrophy of the optical nerve which was cured by smallpox.[14] He also mentioned a personal experience at the Graz Clinic in 1892 when a 19-year-old youth had been brought in with a progressive muscular dystrophy (*Dystrophia musculorum progressiva*). Following a 17-day stay in the Clinic he contracted 'typhus abdominalis', from which he later recovered. During convalescence it was found that the symptoms which had led to his admission to the clinic were gradually disappearing, and he was ultimately discharged as completely cured.

Wagner-Jauregg drew attention to the achievements of 'modern' bacteriology which had shed new light on the different effects of fever on psychoses. He wondered whether this could be explained by the different properties of bacterial toxins, on the one hand, or bacterial proteins, on the other. Whatever the mechanism, Wagner-Jauregg thought that the fact that the effect of fever on psychoses had been documented, challenged the physician to seize the chance of recovery that nature sometimes produced accidentally. There had already been attempts to effect cures by generating feverish conditions, including the use of such therapeutic procedures to bring about and maintain chronic suppuration, as the seton, vesicants, and Autenrieth's ointment. The last procedure was revived with some success by Ludwig Meyer (1827–1900) in cases of *Dementia paralytica*.[15] Over the course of 15 years Meyer treated 17 paralytics by rubbing the ointment on a patch of scalp that had been shaved at least twice, thus causing suppuration. Of these, eight were cured, and their case histories were described in some detail. Wagner-Jauregg was reluctant to use such a drastic procedure. Besides, he could not see why the ointment should have to be applied to the head and not to some less sensitive part of the body if the bacterial infection were indeed the agent of the curative effect.

A little known psychiatrist from Odessa, Alexander S. Rosenblum (1826–1902), for 20 years Chief of Staff of the Odessa Psychopathic Hospital, seems to have been the first to induce a real infectious disease in mental patients. During Wagner-Jauregg's lifetime nothing was known about him in the West, except Oks's reports on Rosenblum's observations and experiments on the effect of fever on psychoses.[16] However, in 1943 S.J. Zakon, prompted by remarks by the American psychiatrist C.A. Neyman, succeeded not only in finding out the salient facts about Rosenblum's life, but also his original article, published in an obscure Odessa journal, entitled

'Relation of febrile diseases to the psychoses', which Zakon translated into English.[17] In it, Rosenblum analysed the literature on the subject and gave an account of the beneficial and curative effects of malaria, typhoid, and recurrent fever on psychoses from his own observations. He studied 22 psychiatric patients, of whom eleven were completely cured after an attack of recurrent fever and three partially cured; the condition of eight remained unchanged. However, in this article Rosenblum did not say that he had induced the fever, although this is clear from his communication to Oks, probably because he feared that in the prevailing political circumstances in Russia this would have met with severe disapproval. From a reading of Oks's paper, Wagner-Jauregg originally considered Rosenblum's experiments to have been the first successful attempts at using feverish illnesses to cure mental illness, and he believed that a report by the bacteriologist Motschutkoffsky from Odessa on recurrent fevers being caused by inoculations[18] might have referred to the same experiments. Later he voiced his doubts as to whether the fevers were induced for therapeutic purposes for the mentally ill and wondering whether this had been done to test the transference of recurrent fevers instead.[19] However, he must have finally reverted to his original view, for he assured V.E. Gonda, whom he met at the International Neurological Congress in London in 1935, that he gave Rosenblum full credit for his daring undertaking.[20]

EXPERIMENTS WITH TUBERCULIN

Not long after the disappointing results Wagner-Jauregg had had with the streptococci inoculations, one of his colleagues and a friend from his Graz days, Theodor Escherich, brought from Berlin a few bottles of tuberculin. One of these he gave to Wagner-Jauregg, who was looking for a safe method of continuing his tests and, as he had written in his 1895 paper,[21] thought that in tuberculin he had found just that. It provided a method for producing artificially the effects of bacterial infection, above all fever, without the dangers of a real bacterial infection. During the winter of 1890/91 he treated a number of patients with favourable results, two of his patients being quickly cured of their psychoses. Nevertheless, he abandoned his experiments for a time. The reason he gave was that cures produced with therapeutic tuberculin were very slow, but at the Graz Clinic only acute cases were admitted and patients were kept only for a short time, so that it was not possible for him to observe the results of the treatment. On the other hand, in his *Memoirs*[22] he confessed that, despite the favourable results he had had with tuberculin, he discontinued his experiments because of alarming reports that the dangers of the therapeutic use of tuberculin had been underestimated and there had even been some deaths as a result.

Robert Koch had claimed that the substance which he had discovered had the power to prevent the growth of tubercle bacilli and that he had had excellent results in clinical trials. However, mounting evidence of the drug's toxicity – particularly Virchow's post-mortem demonstrations of intense local inflammatory reactions in treated cases[23] – intensified doubts about the new remedy. Although Koch had cautioned that only early cases responded at all well, the attack upon him rapidly gained momentum. The *Gazette de Bruxelles* accused him of publishing a 'most audacious and hopeful report' and in July 1891 the Second Congress on Tuberculosis in Paris decided that tuberculin was of very doubtful value.[24] Within twelve months of its introduction, tuberculin passed into a period of profound disrepute. A very vivid description of its over-enthusiastic reception and the dire consequences was given by Theodor Brugsch 1878–1963 in his autobiography.[25] When he was about nine years old he was often taken on walks past a building that was being converted into a coffee house and restaurant. Suddenly it became a tuberculosis sanatorium. No sooner had it been equipped and filled with patients, than he saw hearse after hearse stopping outside the building to carry away the dead. Wagner-Jauregg's two different explanations for discontinuing his tuberculin experiments may well have been due to his reluctance to add his voice to the accusations levelled against Koch.

Soon after Wagner-Jauregg took up his position as Director of the First Clinic in 1893, one of his assistants, Dr Ernst Boeck, wished to test the curative effect of feverish infectious diseases on insanity by injecting bacterial proteins. However, Wagner-Jauregg advised the use of tuberculin instead. It was easily obtainable and he felt that by then sufficient experience had been gained of safe dosages to prevent adverse effects. Consequently, Boeck continued the experiments which Wagner-Jauregg had initiated at Graz of injecting tuberculin into psychiatric patients. He reported on these in 1895.[26] Thirty-three patients were treated, but there were few remissions. Only one among those treated was suffering from GPI. Boeck also injected eight patients with dead cultures of *Bacillus pyocyaneus*, but again the results were disappointing. In this case, unlike that of tuberculin, it was not possible to increase the initial dose.

In a preliminary report on the experiments carried out in collaboration with Boeck[27], Wagner-Jauregg was the more optimistic of the two about the prospects of the treatment. He illustrated the astonishing improvement that could occur with the case of one of his patients who was visited by her sister on the day after the injection. The visitor approached one of the doctors with the question 'What have you done with my sister, she has suddenly become intelligent?' In the same lecture Wagner-Jauregg considered the theoretical problem of whether the fever alone had a curative effect, in which case it would not matter whether tuberculin or some other bacterial protein was injected. If, however, the curative effect depended on the specific characteristics of the bacterial proteins, then a case which failed to respond to treatment with tuberculin might be favourably affected by another bacterial protein. He thought that Boeck had taken the first step in this direction by using dead cultures of *Bacillus pyocyaneus*. Wagner-Jauregg warned his listeners that, although there had been some favourable results, there had also been failures. Nevertheless, he concluded that 'we cannot be reproached for using a procedure which is irrational. We have listened to nature; we have attempted to imitate the method by which nature itself produces cures.'[28]

Wagner-Jauregg continued his experiments with tuberculin after Boeck left the Clinic to take up another appointment. He treated several patients suffering from GPI who responded favourably, and from then on he concentrated his efforts on patients afflicted by that illness. In the postscript to the 1895 paper, published in the collection of his papers,[29] he stated as the reason for this decision that it had been noticeable that among those who had benefited from the tuberculin treatment, there were many more paralytics than patients suffering from other forms of mental illness. Moreover, GPI was thought to be incurable and consequently it could not be said that the patient might have recovered without treatment. Of course, although the clinical diagnosis of GPI was relatively certain, it was not completely reliable until the development of the Wassermann test* in 1906. During the years 1900–1901 Wagner-Jauregg treated 69 cases of patients suffering from GPI with tuberculin and compared them with 69 untreated cases.[30] He worked with dosages of 1 mg to 10 mg. After three years he arranged for his assistant, Dr A. Pilcz, to publish the results.[31] They clearly showed that there were more remissions among the patients who had been treated than among those not subjected to treatment. An

---

* A serological test for syphilis developed by August von Wassermann (1866–1925).

interesting feature of the trial was that the treatment was most beneficial to those whose reaction to the tuberculin was strongest.

Wagner-Jauregg gave an account of his experiments at the Sixteenth International Medical Congress in Budapest in 1909.[32] He had chosen patients in the early stages of paralysis and combined the tuberculin therapy with a treatment with mercury (the standard treatment for syphilis) and iodine, since it had been more or less established by 1902 that GPI was of syphilitic origin.[33] The results of the combined therapy was favourable, many patients making a good recovery and often being able to resume their professional activities. Among patients who did not respond to this treatment a repetition of the therapy often brought favourable results. Forestalling the criticism that there were only remissions but no cure, he argued that this was of little importance because in no field of pathology did the possibility of a recurrence of the illness prevent one from speaking of a cure. In his *Memoirs*, recalling the occasion,[34] he wrote with some irony that the success of his lecture was 'not overwhelming' – in fact, he encountered general scepticism and there was no discussion. Nevertheless, in Vienna at least, the number of unexpected cures of patients suffering from GPI was beginning to attract attention. Wagner-Jauregg also received support from Ernst Meyer (1871–1931), who reported encouraging results after treating 20 paralytic patients with tuberculin and antisyphilitic medication.[35]

A further trial involving 86 patients was made using a combination of tuberculin and mercury and iodine treatment, on which Pilcz reported in 1911[36] and Wagner-Jauregg in 1912.[37] It was found that of 86 patients 23 could be said to be cured and were able to return to their work; 9, although intellectually weak and unable to resume their occupations, were able to return to their families and lead a reasonably normal life; in 20 cases, although there was no essential improvement, the progress of the paralysis was halted; and in the remaining 34 cases the treatment had no effect, the few remissions being short-lived. The patients involved in this trial were in an early stage of paralysis. Because the successive treatments with tuberculin followed by antiluetic agents took some time, a method of applying each on alternate days was adopted.

Two years later Wagner-Jauregg summed up the results of the tuberculin treatment in conjunction with antiluetic medication.[38] He was very critical of the author of the chapter on progressive paralysis in Aschaffenburg's *Handbuch der Psychiatrie*, who did not even mention the tuberculin treatment, but he welcomed the approving papers by E. Meyer and Friedländer,[39] who both quoted favourable results from the treatment. There were also a few other reports on the beneficial effects of the therapy. Speaking of the methodology of the experiments, Wagner-Jauregg said that he much regretted not being able to carry out comparative trials. His hope that these might be undertaken by the asylums, which had a large number of patients whom they were able to observe for a long period, had not been fulfilled. He himself was no longer able to carry out such trials since in 1902, on succeeding Krafft-Ebing, he had exchanged the Clinic at the Asylum for the more important and prestigious Clinic at the General Hospital, where patients were seldom kept for any length of time. The former had no special department for nervous diseases, whereas at the General Hospital there were a Clinic and an Outpatient Department for Nervous Diseases, and consequently a greater variety of cases.

Around 1910, Wagner-Jauregg had decided to experiment with dead cultures of staphylococci using polyvalent preparations made from at least six cultures. He reported on these in 1913.[40] He had treated 39 men suffering from GPI, of whom 23 experienced a distinct remission. Although in 16 the remission was temporary, with the remaining seven it had already lasted for two years. Most of the patients treated suffered from the manic type of paralysis, but Wagner-Jauregg could not say at the time whether such patients had a better chance of a cure. In the collection of his papers on fever therapy, published in 1936,[41] there is a postscript to this paper, the last that appeared before he embarked on his malaria therapy, in which he wrote that he had still been dissatisfied with the results of the treatment that he had pioneered. Although there was a considerable number of complete remissions, they only lasted in a minority of cases; the majority of patients relapsed, even though they were able to resume their occupation for a year or two. The best results occurred when some feverish illness intervened. This circumstance suggested to him to produce in paralytics a real infectious disease, the course of which could be controlled and which would not endanger the environment.

MALARIA THERAPY

As early as 1887, Wagner-Jauregg had suggested the artificial production of tertian malaria. A chance event caused him to take up the idea, and this led to the beginning of malaria therapy in June 1917. There is a vivid account of this event in his *Memoirs*.[42] One of his colleagues, Dr Alfred Fuchs, reported to him that a soldier who had been admitted to hospital on his return from the Macedonian front with a slight injury to his nerves was suffering attacks of fever, accompanied by shivering fits of the tertiana type, and asked whether he ought to give him quinine. Immediately, the idea occurred to Wagner-Jauregg to inoculate GPI sufferers with the blood of this malaria patient. 'No', he replied to his colleague, and he explained what he intended to do.

So on 14 June 1917 he took blood from the vein of the soldier during an attack of fever and inoculated two paralytics with it. Then he became worried lest there were some anopheles mosquitoes in the grounds of the Clinic and the malaria might spread. He got one of the neurotic patients who was still able to carry out simple tasks to catch as many gnats as he could and bring them in for examination. To his great relief there were no anopheles mosquitoes among them. Thus encouraged, he took blood twice more from the malaria patient and injected it subcutaneously under the skin of the back of paralytic patients. From the blood of the GPI patients who contracted malaria in this way three more patients were infected by subcutaneous injection, and with the blood of one of this group two more patients were injected. In all these cases the presence of tertian plasmodium was microscopically confirmed in the blood.

At the invitation of the editor of the *Psychiatrisch-neurologische Wochenschrift*, Wagner-Jauregg gave a detailed account of the case histories of the first nine patients treated with malaria.[43] Apart from one patient who died while Wagner-Jauregg was away on a scientific medical commission to the Isonzo front and two who had to be sent to the Asylum after a few months, the remaining six all showed considerable improvement, but all except two eventually suffered relapses. Of the latter, one was a tram conductor, 34 years old, who had joined the army in 1915. He was admitted to the Clinic as insane early in June 1917. After eleven attacks of fever he was treated with quinine. His improvement was slow but steady. He recovered, and a little more than a year after admission was sent back to his regiment for auxiliary duties at his own request. The other was a clerical worker, 39 years old, suffering from the manic type of general paralysis. After he had had ten attacks of fever he was treated with quinine and later with salvarsan. He recovered completely and was able to resume his work.

Of the remaining four who were discharged as cured and able to resume their work, one, a woman cleaner, had to be re-admitted the following year. Another, a railway worker, who left the Clinic about a year after the treatment, later committed suicide in a state of depression. In the third case, that of a sergeant-major admitted in the manic state of paralysis, the remission only lasted for a few months. The story of the fourth, actually the first to be treated, is extraordinary. The patient was a 37-year-old actor who was admitted to the Clinic suffering from loss of memory and epileptic fits due to suspected paralysis. As a result of the malaria treatment he improved so much that within two months he was able to give performances at social evenings for patients. He was discharged at the end of the year and was able to resume his profession. In a postscript to the paper, added in 1936,[44] Wagner-Jauregg recounted how some months later he received an enquiry from Dr Raphael Weichbrodt (b. 1886) of the Frankfurt-am-Main Asylum regarding this patient, who had evidently had a relapse. His wife had told Dr Weichbrodt of the miraculously successful treatment that her husband had received in Vienna, and of course Dr Weichbrodt wanted to know more about it. When Wagner-Jauregg wrote to him about the malaria therapy (he had not published anything at that time), Weichbrodt inoculated four of his paralytic patients with malaria and had great success with two of them. He later used inoculations with spirilla causing recurrent fever.

In all the cases that Wagner-Jauregg treated with malaria, he administered, after seven to twelve attacks of fever, 1 g of quinine bisulphate a day for three days and then 0.5 g daily for fourteen days. In each case the fever ceased after the first few doses. In addition, the patients received three intravenous injections of neosalvarsan at weekly intervals. It was noticed that in most cases the fever attacks turned into the quotidian type.

Wagner-Jauregg was keen to continue his trials of malaria therapy. Since he had no malaria patients at his Clinic, he approached a specialist in internal medicine, who was in charge of a department in a military hospital where there were many malaria patients, to let him have blood from a confirmed case of tertian malaria.[45] Unfortunately, he omitted to examine microscopically the blood received (fearing that any delay might affect the infectious nature of the blood) and he immediately injected one paralytic patient with it. When this patient's temperature began to rise, he took blood from him and injected three other paralytic patients with it. The first patient became seriously ill; the fever did not cease despite large doses of quinine. The blood test showed that nearly all his blood cells were covered with plasmodia. The number of red corpuscles decreased frighteningly and the white cells disappeared altogether. It was clearly a malignant type of *malaria tropica*. The patient died after 31 days, as did two others who had been injected. The fourth survived after large doses of quinine and neosalvarsan were administered for 45 days; his paralysis was cured completely and lastingly. Nevertheless, the fate that befell the other patients discouraged Wagner-Jauregg and he did not feel able to continue his trials with malaria, particularly as some authorities claimed to be able to achieve better results with injections of spirilla causing recurrent fever.

It was a year before he resumed his trials, when the bacteriologist Professor R. Doerr (1871–1952) came to his aid. He had found a case of confirmed tertian malaria. The patient lived in an area where autochthonous cases of malaria occasionally occurred. Often there were malaria cases among the crew of the steamers which brought goods to Vienna from Hungary, Serbia, Romania and Bulgaria. The inhabitants on both banks of the Danube sometimes became infected if they were bitten by an anopheles mosquito that had previously attacked one of the sailors. Although Doerr was not concerned with the fate of the paralytic patients, he needed to make experiments with malaria vaccination, and at his request three paralytic patients were injected with different concentrations of the blood from the malaria patient. In his *Memoirs* Wagner-Jauregg reported that the 'results of the experiments did not come up to Professor Doerr's expectations',[46] because it was not the patient who had received the strongest concentration of the blood who developed malaria, but the one who was given one of medium strength. Wagner-Jauregg decided to make no more experiments with different concentrations, particularly because in the meantime Doerr had left Vienna to take up an appointment in Basle. From the paralytic patient who received blood from Doerr's malaria patient in September 1919 blood was taken to vaccinate further paralytic patients in a continual passage from one to another. From this time the malaria therapy of progressive paralysis was continued at the Vienna Psychiatric Clinic on a large scale without interruption. All patients suffering from GPI, both men and women, and also those suffering from tabes were treated. More and more patients who had come to the Clinic as hopeless cases were able to return to their families and their work, and more and more sufferers came to the Clinic to be treated.

It so happened that Wagner-Jauregg was chosen as a representative of Austria on the Council of the German Society for Psychiatry. In the autumn of 1920 its Annual Conference took place in Hamburg, and among the speakers was a physician from the Hamburg Municipal Asylum who reported on behalf of three colleagues on the results they had achieved in an attempt to treat GPI by inoculation with tertian and tropical malaria. Only at the end of this communication did the speaker mention that Wagner-Jauregg had made similar experiments. When the lecture was published in the *Münchner Medizinische Wochenschrift* two months after the meeting,[47] Wagner-Jauregg's priority was acknowledged. In his reply Wagner-Jauregg stressed that he had carried out the first inoculations with malaria in 1917, but had discontinued them for one year to await results. (In fact, as mentioned above, he had interrupted his experiments for a time because he had become discouraged as a result of the disastrous consequences of the use of *malaria tropica* instead of *tertiana*.) After resuming his treatments, Wagner-Jauregg said, he had achieved many more cures than the three workers mentioned. He was, however, able to warn them against the use of *malaria tropica*. In a lecture in February 1921[48] Wagner-Jauregg said that more than 150 cases had received the malaria treatment, and more than a dozen had been able to resume work. In some cases the remission had lasted for more than three years. Later that year[49] he reported that more than 200 patients had been treated, of whom 50 had been able to return to work.

A more detailed account of the treatments and the results achieved was given by J. Gerstmann (b. 1887), one of the assistants at Wagner-Jauregg's Clinic, in two articles published in 1920 and 1922 and in book form in 1925.[50] By that time the number of paralytics treated exceeded 1000. Although at first very advanced cases of paralysis were not subjected to the malaria therapy, during the last two years under review all paralytics admitted to the Clinic were so treated. However, in the statistical analysis only fully or partially successful cases that had been observed for two years or more were included, i.e. 400 cases. Over 60 per cent of the patients experienced remissions of different degrees.

Gerstmann related the fascinating case histories of five patients who made a complete recovery. They were middle-aged men, three in clerical occupations, one an upholsterer and one a driver. They were all brought to the Clinic with various symptoms of progressive paralysis and all had contracted a syphilitic infection several years previously. They showed impairment of mental functions and speech, besides symptoms such as megalomania, mania, euphoria, paralytic seizures. They were treated with tertian malaria, the onset of a remission varying greatly from patient to patient. It was often some time before an improvement was noted. In one case it took two months, in another the patient was returned to the asylum as he showed no sign of recovery, but his condition gradually improved so much that he was able to take up his previous post after six months. The other patients recovered gradually after the attacks of fever.

Needless to say, early cases of paralysis had a much higher chance of recovery than those who had suffered from the disease for some years. In cases of long standing, it was to be expected that GPI had caused irreversible changes in the nervous system. The two symptoms that were most regularly improved by the therapy were defects of speech and writing. It was remarkable how patients whose writing was jittery and uncoordinated reverted to normality in this respect. Patients who had suffered paralytic seizures also responded well to the treatment. On the other hand, even in cases of complete recovery, pupil reactions did not return to normal. Moreover, it was usually some time before the Wassermann reaction of the serum and spinal fluid became negative.

In a talk Wagner-Jauregg gave to general practitioners in 1922,[51] he outlined the use of tuberculin therapy in conjunction with mercury or neosalvarsan treatment for paralytics, some time after this had been replaced by malaria therapy with its far superior results. This was probably because the latter could only be carried out in hospitals, whereas the former was available to practitioners. He gave full details of the dosages he advocated and the method of injecting. He also suggested the use of typhus vaccine both in GPI and tabes.

In view of the favourable results obtained in early cases of paralysis and the fact that it was known who might succumb to the disease – those who having contracted syphilis some time previously still had positive Wassermann reactions – it seemed advisable to treat these patients before the onset of paralysis. One of Wagner-Jauregg's assistants, Dr Bernhard Dattner, suggested that this ought to be done, but there were no patients of this kind at the Clinic.[52] They were to be found at the Clinic for Syphilis and therefore Wagner-Jauregg sent Dattner to Professor Josef Kyrle (1880–1926) there with this suggestion. Kyrle was at first unwilling for them to be treated, maintaining that it was one thing to inoculate with malaria a paralytic who was a hopeless case and quite another to treat a seemingly healthy person in this way just because his reaction was positive. However, a few weeks later, Kyrle told Wagner-Jauregg that he had tried the treatment and it had worked. He reported on his work at a joint meeting of the German Society for Psychiatry and the Society of German Neurologists and Venereologists in September 1924.[53] Wagner-Jauregg described experiments to prove whether, and under what conditions, induced malaria could be transmitted by the anopheles mosquito. They were carried out by the Italian bacteriologist Dr G. Barzillai-Vivaldi and were performed at Wagner-Jauregg's Clinic, with the assistance of Dr O. Kauders (1893–1949) between June and August 1924. These complicated experiments involved the use of a large number of *Anopheles maculi pennis*, which had been bred in Rome. The insects were distributed in cages covered with netting through which they were able to bite a number of paralytic patients who were suffering from malaria fever at different stages of severity. Later six paralytic patients who had not yet been subjected to the malaria therapy were brought into the same room. They too were exposed to bites from these mosquitoes so that they should be infected with malaria. Altogether they suffered 127 bites. After three weeks not one of these six patients had been infected. They were later subjected to the malaria therapy which followed its usual course. The experiments proved that induced malaria could not be transmitted by anopheles bite.

MALARIA THERAPY WORLD-WIDE

It was not long after Wagner-Jauregg published details of his malaria therapy that the treatment was introduced at the Hamburg Asylum and the Hamburg Clinic for Nervous Diseases. During 1920 several other institutions in Germany followed suit. By 1921 the treatment had been introduced in the Netherlands and South America; by 1922 it had spread to Britain, Italy and Czechoslovakia and by 1923 its use was reported in the United States, Russia, Denmark and France. During the following years, 1924, 1925 and 1926 there were many reports on the use of malaria therapy at institutions all over the world. In the Index Catalogue to the Surgeon General's Library (4th series, Volume 8), published in Washington in 1929, there are three closely printed columns listing papers, published in the mid-1920s, on malaria therapy in the treatment of GPI. Most of these articles leave no doubt that Wagner-Jauregg's discovery was welcomed and appreciated. The descriptions used were 'a therapeutic noble deed', 'a distinct advance in treatment', 'the right way to treat a hopeless disease', 'unquestionably a method of value', 'the best treatment available'. A. Hoche (1865–1943) in Switzerland thought it a duty to use the malaria treatment.[54] As early as 1923 an Editorial in the *American Journal of Psychiatry* urged that observations be made on the effects of malarial infection on the progress of paresis. 'It may be that every large hospital for mental disorders may have to maintain one or more malarial patients as source of infectious material.'[55] In Britain, too, there were favourable comments. An Editorial in *Nature* urged that every endeavour should be made to investigate and perfect a method that offered hope of improvement.[56] Warrington Yorke, commenting on results achieved at a number of mental hospitals in the Liverpool area, called them remarkable.[57] Henry R. Rollin, in his recently published autobiography, describes how Wagner-Jauregg's therapy was begun at the Horton Hospital in Epsom on 25 May 1925 when mosquitoes infected with a strain of parasite provided by the Horton Malaria Laboratory were fed on two women GPI patients.[58] The Laboratory provided material for many thousands of victims of GPI in hospitals in Britain, including some 16 000 in Horton alone, until penicillin made this treatment obsolete. The reception of the therapy was particularly enthusiastic in the United States, where it was adopted in many institutions, including the New York State Psychiatric Institute, and asylums at Madison (Wisconsin), Indianapolis and Harrisburg.

The results were broadly consistent. Generally, the success rate was about 30 per cent full remission and 20 per cent partial remission. Most reports agreed that the Wassermann reaction of the serum and spinal fluid remained positive for a considerable time and did not always revert to normal. In such cases, Wagner-Jauregg recommended, the malaria treatment should be repeated.[59]

The mode of infecting the patient varied from country to country. In Britain, instead of producing the disease by the inoculation of malaria blood, it was sometimes induced by the bite of infected mosquitoes. Three American researchers also reported better results when the patient was infected directly by a mosquito, rather than inoculated with infected blood.[60] Wagner-Jauregg was not in favour of the former method, which involved true, not induced malaria. He thought that the latter responded more readily to treatment with quinine and did not recur afterwards. He recommended the use of blood that was free from trypanosome gametes; this offered much better protection for the environment.[61]

Some German researchers used the African recurrent fever in place of malaria and obtained good results. Wagner-Jauregg speaking of the differences between these two types of treatment, said that recurrent fever caused an immunity, the duration of which could not be gauged, and this treatment, unlike malaria, could therefore not be repeated. Moreover, it was impossible to stop the fever attacks because they did not respond to treatment with quinine. At Wagner-Jauregg's Clinic a comparative trial was made for four months during the spring and summer of 1925 in which one patient was treated with malaria, the next with recurrent fever and so on. Of 33 patients treated with malaria 14 recovered from general paralysis and were able to return to their professions and 10 showed incomplete remissions; whereas of the 33 treated with recurrent fever only 6 recovered and 9 showed incomplete remissions. In Wagner-Jauregg's view, the European and American types of recurrent fever were too dangerous to consider as a possible treatment. The most effective method of treatment was induced malaria, particularly if it was combined with specific treatment with salvarsan.[62]

In an appreciation of Wagner-Jauregg's work on the 90th anniversary of his birth, one of his former assistants, O. Kauders (later head of the Clinic), spoke of the different methods examined, such as recurrent fever, rat-bite fever and quartan malaria. He emphasised that Wagner-Jauregg did not make the tests himself, but let others carry them out so that the results would be unprejudiced. Wagner-Jauregg was always ready to abandon his own method in favour of a better one and was not blind to the faults of his achievement. He always insisted on controlled trials, which he termed *Simultan Methode*.[63]

In a report which he was invited to give at the 38th Congress of the German Society for Internal Medicine, in Wiesbaden in 1926, on the modern treatment of neuro-syphilis,[64] he gave a detailed account of contemporary efforts at treating the disease and summarised his own researches over the previous years. He discussed experiments and facts which offered some explanation of the effect of treatment with malaria and recurrent fever. He believed that the fever produced by malaria should not be regarded as the principal cause of the therapeutic effect, because although the temperatures induced by recurrent fever or tuberculin were considerably lower, yet treatment with them had been effective. No spirochaetes were found in the brains of paralytics who, before their deaths, underwent an illness accompanied by high fever.

In concluding his report, Wagner-Jauregg emphasised that both malaria and the African recurrent fever had proved far the most effective methods, not only of treating GPI, but also in prophylactic treatment – that is in procuring negative results in the analysis of spinal fluid. As far as the treatment of tabes was concerned, these methods could also be recommended with certain provisos. As Wagner-Jauregg wrote in his 1926 paper on neurolues,[65] tabes presented different problems from those of GPI. The latter followed a rapid and increasingly malignant course, but inclined to considerable remissions requiring quick intervention, whereas tabes progressed much more slowly and had inconsiderable remissions, but sometimes remained stationary for unlimited periods. In the case of GPI drastic treatment was necessary, whereas a patient suffering from tabes who walked with two sticks could still be a useful member of society. However, the treatment of tabes with malaria had to be applied with caution and be limited to the preataxic stages of the disease. In the early stages of the disease it could have excellent results.

In four papers published respectively in 1924 (two), 1926 and 1927,[66] Wagner-Jauregg dealt with some of the symptoms of tabes. In the first, on the stabbing pains of tabes sufferers, he speculated on their cause. He believed them to be due to changes in nerve fibres, similar to those after operations. The second paper dealt with tabic diseases of the joints which affect mostly the lower extremities. In the third paper Wagner-Jauregg discussed gastric crises in tabes sufferers and their treatment. The fourth paper in this series, based on a lecture to the Vienna Ophthalmological Society, is much more extensive. In it, he reviewed at some length the work of several researchers on optic atrophy in tabes. As far as treatment with malaria was concerned, the prognosis was less favourable than in GPI.

Wagner-Jauregg embarked on his researches on the effect of fever on psychoses in 1887 and he first experimented on producing fever in 1888/89. Thirty years were to elapse before in 1917 he began his work on the use of malaria for treating paralytics. He had to wait many years for recognition of his achievements. In 1926 he was awarded the Erb-medal of the Society of German Neurologists and was made an Honorary Member of that Society. In 1927 the

German Society for Psychiatry moved the venue of their annual meeting to Vienna in his honour and bestowed Honorary Membership on him; in the same year he was awarded the Nobel Prize. His name had been put forward for the prize as early as 1924 but, according to Wagner-Jauregg, the referee at the time, B. Gadelius (1862–1938), a Swedish Professor of Psychiatry, could not be persuaded to recommend the award to 'a physician who injected malaria into a paralytic, because he was in his eyes a criminal'. So Wagner-Jauregg had to wait until Gadelius retired. Copies of the documents concerning the award to Wagner-Jauregg, which were kindly made available to the author by the Nobel Committee, do not reveal why Wagner-Jauregg did not receive the award in 1924. However, the Secretary of the Nobel Committee has confirmed that Gadelius ceased to be a member of the Committee on 31 December 1925.

In his *Memoirs* Wagner-Jauregg told how he received news of the award of the prize.[67] The decision on the proposed candidates was usually taken at the end of September. Wagner-Jauregg had seen a notice in one of the Vienna daily papers regarding the prospective candidates for the award of the prize in medicine, but his name was not among these and he had therefore resigned himself to the fact that he would not receive the prize. One evening at about 10 o'clock in September 1927 he was telephoned by a Berlin newspaper, asking whether he knew that he was among the candidates: he denied any knowledge and the journalist rang again an hour later to say that the meeting of the Karoline Institute was still in session. He thereupon went to bed and went to sleep, only to be re-awakened at one o'clock by another telephone call from the same Berlin correspondent who told him that he had been awarded the Nobel Prize. There was no question of sleep after that and he did what he often did when he could not sleep: he got up and played chess against himself, following some master match from a chess tournament. Early the following morning he received a telephone call from Stockholm advising him of the award of the Nobel Prize. In an article in the *Illustrierte Zeitung* of Leipzig written in the year of his death at the age of 83, in which he gave a short account of the malaria therapy, he said that the malaria therapy was his most important work. It brought many men cure of an illness that had until then been considered incurable. It also brought him not only many honours and awards, but – what was more important for him – personal satisfaction in the days of old age.

Even after Wagner-Jauregg had received the Nobel Prize for his malaria therapy he did not rest on his laurels, but continued his investigations on various aspects of the treatment. One that troubled him was the reason why malaria tertiana often turned into the quotidian type. In an article in 1927[68] he said that more experiments were needed to examine whether it was the method of injecting or the constitution of the patient that was responsible. This was important because, in treating paralytics, the change from tertian to quotidian malaria was an embarrassment because the latter did not allow the patient enough time to recover from the fever. In a subsequent paper on the significance of blood groups for induced malaria,[69] he considered the effect of the relation of the blood groups between the person from whom blood is taken and the person who receives it. This had been examined by Wethmar who also investigated the effect of the method of injection. He found that a favourable relation between blood groups of donor and recipient (non-agglutinating) and intravenous injection resulted in more quotidian types than an agglutinating relation and subcutaneous injection.[70] The reason for this seems to be the differential development of the plasmodia.

A much later paper on the danger of therapeutic malaria spreading to the environment[71] was an attempt to deal with criticisms by E. Martini (b. 1880),[72] who argued against the use of induced malaria. Wagner-Jauregg claimed that more than 3000 patients had received the malaria treatment and that there had not been one case of malaria among the medical staff. There were no cases of infection in two Berlin institutions and only two cases had been reported from Sweden and one from Göttingen. Martini saw the greatest danger in cases of recurring malaria, but Wagner-Jauregg tried to show that no such cases were observed in Vienna, nor reported from other clinics, where sufficient doses of quinine had been used.

In an article on the optimum effect of malaria therapy, Wagner-Jauregg again stressed the desirability of early treatment of GPI.[73] The earlier it was initiated, the greater the probability of remission. It was obvious therefore that the results of treatment of patients in clinics for nervous diseases were far better than for those in asylums. He believed that the optimum number of malaria attacks before stopping them with quinine was eight. If the patient was not fit enough to withstand so many, it was wise to interrupt the treatment after four attacks and then repeat the therapy four to six weeks later. Wagner-Jauregg also recommended this method of treatment when the patient was either too fat or too emaciated, or if he suffered from some other disease. The malaria treatment had to be followed by a specific therapy, usually neosalvarsan and bismogenol or tryparsamid as used in America. In cases promising complete remission no further treatment was required, but Wagner-Jauregg recommended that doubtful cases should undergo a second malaria cure and that malaria therapy should also be repeated if the lumbar puncture result, i.e. the result of the Wassermann test of the spinal fluid for the presence of syphilitic infection, was still positive after six months.

Wagner-Jauregg was always ready to consider criticisms of his malaria therapy and to examine alternative methods of treatment. He discussed at some length the use of short-wave high frequency currents and the advantages and disadvantages of this procedure.[74] Infections from the blood donor to the recipient were avoided by this treatment, but it involved much discomfort. Wagner-Jauregg refuted the assumption that the effect of the malaria therapy was due mainly to the high temperature reached and its duration, because complete remission of GPI had been achieved with fever temperatures well below those necessary for the destruction of the spirochaetes. In Vienna it was not possible to test the radiothermal and diathermal treatments as there were no funds to buy the equipment, but those in charge were happy with the results of the malaria therapy which was cheap. The principal reason for the success of the malaria therapy was not its effect on the organism causing the paralysis, but the increased resistance which the nervous system developed to react to the syphilitic infection.[75]

Wagner-Jauregg emphasised this point of view in some letters to Paul de Kruif,[76] the author of *Men Against Death*,[77] drafts of which were found among the documents he left. He seemed inordinately pleased with the chapter on him and his malaria therapy in that book, a copy of which was sent to him by the author. In expressing his thanks, in a letter dated April 1933, he said that de Kruif had erected a literary monument which would outlast him. He referred to the chapter on 'Infektions- und Fiebertherapy' for Volume 8 of the *Handbuch der Neurologie*[78] as probably his swan song. He promised to send an offprint to de Kruif.

In a letter dated August 1935 to de Kruif, Wagner-Jauregg

171

apologised for the delay in replying to de Kruif's letter of 3 September 1934, saying that it was due to the same slowness in decision that was responsible for the slow progress from the tuberculin to the malaria therapy. He now had a good reason for writing, because he was posting under separate cover a lecture in English[79] which he had prepared for the members of the Academic Senate and the Professorial Board of the University of Edinburgh, as he was unable for health reasons to travel to Edinburgh to receive the Cameron prize for 1935 which had been awarded to him for his malaria therapy. In the same letter he expressed his surprise how quickly his therapy had taken root in America and how many different methods of producing fever had been developed in that country. He referred to the excellent results obtained with a combination of high-frequency and tryparsamid therapy and regretted that it was too costly to be applied generally in Austria. At his Clinic results had become disappointing because most cases of GPI now were those in an advanced state of the disease, victims of early GPI having been treated at clinics for syphilis and in other hospital departments.

As late as 1939, a year before his death, Wagner-Jauregg at the age of 82 described in great detail the state of the treatment of GPI.[80] He thought that the time had come to consider whether his malaria therapy was still the most efficient treatment, or whether chemotherapy or the production of high temperatures by physical means could claim to be as good or even better. At the Vienna Clinic stress was laid on the need to combine malaria therapy with chemotherapy, for example treatment with 5-valent arsenic preparations, such as tryparsamid which had been developed by the Rockefeller Foundation in America, and Stovarsol by I.G. Farben in Germany. Both these had a very favourable effect on late forms of neurosyphilis, particularly on the spinal fluid. Wagner-Jauregg discussed in detail a number of trials carried out in the United States, comparing different methods of treatment, of which there were three available for producing fever by physical means: (1) the diathermy apparatus; (2) the radiotherm apparatus which produced high temperatures by shortwave high frequency currents; and (3) the Kettering hypertherm apparatus based on the production of superheated humid air. From the data given it seems that a combination of a fever therapy, produced either by malaria or radiotherm, together with chemotherapy, offered the best prospects of remission, but as Wagner-Jauregg pointed out equipment for the latter and its operation were much more costly. The best treatment of GPI remained prophylaxis, that is an energetically carried out chemotherapy, immediately an infection had been diagnosed, with a view to rendering the Wassermann reaction of the spinal fluid negative.

In a letter to his son, dated 29 March 1940,[81] a few months before his death Wagner-Jauregg expressed his concern regarding criticism of the dangers involved in his malaria therapy by Bering of Cologne and E. Hoffmann (1868–1959) of Bonn. However, most of the letter dealt with Bering's attempts at using X-rays in the treatment of GPI. Wagner-Jauregg had a poor opinion of Bering's knowledge of psychiatry and neurology and thought that of the fifteen cases treated by X-rays, on which Bering had reported, half might not have been suffering from GPI. Nevertheless, he said he did not wish to publicise his critisism because he did not want to hurt Bering, who was a friend of his and had supported the malaria therapy in late stages of syphilis. Moreover, Bering was a professor at Cologne and he had no wish to anatagonise the faculty there. In the letter Wagner-Jauregg also asked his son, who was a pharmaceutical chemist, about two preparations used in the treatment of syphilitics and the method of their administration.

In his concluding remarks to the collection of his papers on *Fever and Infection Therapy*, published in 1936,[82] Wagner-Jauregg said that the fever therapy would become redundant if it were possible to treat all cases of syphilitic infection in its early stages with specific means, for example with the tri-valent arsenic preparations. Since most men were too indolent to submit to early treatment, and because of the occurrence of inherited syphilis, this was unlikely to be achieved. Wagner-Jauregg thought that the elimination of syphilis lay in the distant future. Alas, he did not live long enough to see the discovery of antibiotics.

References

[1] L. Schönbauer and M. Jantsch. Ed. Julius Wagner-Jauregg, *Lebenserinnerungen*. Wien: Springer Verlag, 1950, p. 152.

[2] Julius Wagner-Jauregg. Ueber die Einwirkung fieberhafter Erkrankungen auf Psychosen. *Jahrb.Psychiat.Neurol.*, 1887, 7: 94–131.

[3] Wagner-Jauregg, op.cit. ref 2, pp. 98–102.

[4] Wagner-Jauregg, op.cit. ref 2, p. 104.

[5] Wagner-Jauregg, op.cit. ref 2, pp. 107–114.

[6] W. Nasse. Zur Diagnose und Prognose der allgemeinen fortschreitenden Paralyse der Irren. *Irrenfreund*, 1870, 12: 97–115.

M. Gauster. Die Heilung allgemeiner Paralyse. *Jahrb.Psychiat. Neurol.*, 1879, 1: 3–55.

Doutrebente. Pathologie des différentes espèces de remisions qui surviennent dans le cours de la paralysie generale progressive. *Ann.Med.Psychol.*, 1878, 19: 161–180, 321–341.

[7] Wagner-Jauregg, op.cit. ref 2, pp. 121–124.

[8] F. Köstl. *Correspondenzblatt der deutschen Gesellschaft für Psychiatrie*, 1856 (as quoted by Wagner-Jauregg; not confirmed).

J.G. Kiernan. Variola and insanity. *Zentralbl.Nervenheilk.*, 1884, 7: 68 (abstracted from *Am.J.Neurol.Psychiat.*, 1883, 2: 365–372.)

[9] M. Leidesdorf. *Anzeiger der kk. Gesellschaft der Aerzte in Wien*, 1875 (as quoted by Wagner-Jauregg; not confirmed).

[10] B. Oks. Ueber die Wirkung fieberhafter Krankheiten auf Heilung von Psychosen. *Arch.Psychiat.*, 1880, 10: 249–256.

Motschukoffsky. Experimentelle Studien über die Impfbarkeit typhöser Fieber. *Zentralbl.Med.Wiss.*, 1876, 14: no. 11, 193–194.

[11] As a result of Fehleisen's experiments it was possible to produce pure cultures of streptococci.

[12] Julius Wagner-Jauregg. *Lebenserinnerungen.* Ed. L. Schönbauer und M. Jantsch. Wien: Springer Verlag, 1950, p. 157.

[13] Julius Wagner-Jauregg. Psychiatrische Heilbestrebungen. *Wien. Klin.Wschr.*,1895, 8: no. 9, 155–159.

[14] L. Mauthner. Heilpotenzen am Sehorgan. *Wien.Klin.Wschr.*, 1894, 7: 318–319.

[15] L. Meyer. Die Behandlung der allgemeinen progressiven Paralyse (Dementia paralytica). *Berl.Klin.Wschr.*, 1877, 14: no. 21, 289–293.

[16] Oks, op.cit. ref 10.

[17] A.S. Rosenblum. Relation of febrile diseases to the psychoses. *Arch.Derm.Syph.*, 1943, 48: 52–58 (transl. from *Trudi vrach.Odessk. g.boln.*, 1876–1877, vol. 2, pt. B. by S.J. Zakon, with comments by C.A. Neymann).

[18] Motschutkoffsky, op.cit. ref 10.

[19] Julius Wagner-Jauregg. *Fieber- und Infektionstherapie.* Wien: Weidmann und Co., 1936, pp. 74–75.

[20] V.E. Gonda. Wagner-Jauregg and the 'priority' of producing artificial fever for treatment of general paresis. *Am.J.Psychiat. Neurol.*, 1957, 114: 561–562.

[21] Wagner-Jauregg, op.cit. ref 13.

[22] Wagner-Jauregg, op.cit. ref 12.

23 R. Virchow. On the action of Koch's remedy upon internal organs in tuberculosis. *Lancet*, 1891, i, 130–132.

24 A.G. Macintyre. Tuberculin therapy. *Oxford Medical School Gazette*, 1954, 6: 146–152.

25 Th. Brugsch. *Arzt seit fünf Jahrzehnten*. Berlin: Rütten und Loening, 1957.

26 E. Boeck. Versuche über die Einwirkung künstlich erzeugten Fiebers bei Psychosen. *Jahrb.Psychiat.Neurol.*, 1895, 14: 199–268.

27 Wagner-Jauregg, op.cit. ref 13.

28 Ibid., p. 159.

29 Wagner-Jauregg, op.cit. ref 19.

30 Wagner-Jauregg, op.cit. ref 12.

31 A. Pilcz. Ueber Heilversuche an Paralytikern. *Jahrb.Psychiat.Neurol.*, 1905, 25: 141–167.

32 Julius Wagner-Jauregg. Ueber die Behandlung der progressiven Paralyse. *Wien.Med.Wschr.*, 1909, 59: no. 37, 2124–2127.

33 In 1893 J.A. Fournier in *Les affections parasyphilitiques*, Paris: Rueff, 1894, had proposed that there was a causal relation between tabes and general paralysis of the insane with syphilis.
    Actually, as early as 1857 F. Esmarch and W. Jessen in *Allg. Z.Psychiat.*, 1857, 14: 20–36, suggested a connection between general paralysis of the insane and syphilis.

34 Wagner-Jauregg, op.cit. ref 12.

35 E. Meyer. Zur Behandlung der progressiven Paralyse. *Münch. Med.Wschr.*, 1912, no. 49, 2704.

36 A. Pilcz. Zur Prognose und Behandlung der progressiven Paralyse. *Zentralbl.Gesamte Neurol.Psychiat.*, 1911, 4: no. 4; abstract ibid. 3: 94–95.

37 Julius Wagner-Jauregg. Zur Behandlung der progressiven Paralyse mit Bakterientoxinen. *Wien.Klin.Wschr.*, 1912, 25: no. 1, 61–63.

38 Julius Wagner-Jauregg. Die Tuberkulin-Quecksilberbehandlung der progressiven Paralyse. *Therap.Monatshefte*, 1914, 28: 1–8.

39 Meyer, op.cit. ref 35.
    Friedländer. Ueber die Einwirkung fieberhafter Prozesse auf metaluetische Erkrankungen des Zentralnervensystems. *Münch. Med.Wschr.*, 1912, no. 38, 2038–2040.

40 Julius Wagner-Jauregg. Ueber Behandlung der progressiven Paralyse mit Staphylokokkenvakzine. *Wien.Med.Wschr.*, 1913, 63: no. 39, 2556–2558.

41 Wagner-Jauregg, op.cit. ref 19.

42 Wagner-Jauregg, op.cit. ref 12.

43 Julius Wagner-Jauregg. Ueber die Einwirkung der Malaria auf die progressive Paralyse. *Psychiat.Neurol.Wschr.*, 1918, no. 21/22, 132–134; 1919, No. 39/40, 251–255.

44 Wagner-Jauregg, op.cit. ref 19.

45 Wagner-Jauregg, op.cit. ref 12.

46 Ibid p. 166.

47 P. Mühlens, W. Weygandt and W. Kirschbaum. Die Behandlung der Paralyse mit Malaria- und Rekurrensfieber. *Münch.Med.Wschr.*, 1920, 67: 831–833.

48 Julius Wagner-Jauregg. Die Behandlung der progressiven Paralyse und Tabes. *Wien.Med.Wschr.*, 1921, 71: no. 25, 1105–1109; no. 27, 1209–1215.

49 Julius Wagner-Jauregg. The treatment of general paresis by inoculation of malaria. *J.Nerv.Ment.Dis.*, 1922, 55: 369–375.

50 J. Gerstmann. Ueber die Einwirkung der Malaria tertiana auf die progressive Paralyse. *Zentralbl.gesamte Neurol.Psychiat.*, 1920, 60: 328–359; 1922, 74: 242–258; *Die Malariabehandlung der progressiven Paralyse*. Wien: Springer, 1925.

51 Julius Wagner-Jauregg. *Wien.Med.Wschr.*, 1922, 72: no. 1.

52 Wagner-Jauregg, op.cit. ref 12.

53 88. Versammlung Deutscher Naturforscher und Aerzte in Innsbruck. *Zentralbl.gesamte Neurol.Psychiat.*, 1925, 39: 464–480; G. Barzilai Vivaldi und O. Kauders. Die Impfmalaria – experimentell durch Anophelen nicht übertragbar. *Wien.Klin.Wschr.*, 1924, 37: 1055–57.

54 A. Hoche. Die Behandlung der progressiven Paralyse. *Schweiz. Med.Wschr.*, 1925, 6: 133–135.

55 'Editorial'. *Am.J.Psychiat.*, 1923, 79: 721–723.

56 'The malarial treatment of general paralysis'. *Nature*, 1924, 114: 164–165.

57 Warrington Yorke. The malarial treatment of general paresis. *Nature*, 1924, 114: 615.

58 Henry R. Rollin. *Festina Lente, A Psychiatric Odyssey*. London: *British Medical Journal*, 1990, p. 51.

59 Julius Wagner-Jauregg. *Verhandlungen der deutschen Gesellschaft für Innere Medizin*, 38. Congress Wiesbaden, April 1926, pp. 34–62.

60 E. Kusch, D.F. Milam and W.K. Stratman-Thomas. General paresis treated by mosquito inoculated tertian malaria. *Am.J. Psychiat.*, 1936, 93: 619.

61 Wagner-Jauregg, op.cit. ref 59.

62 Wagner-Jauregg, op.cit. ref 59.

[63] O. Kauders. Julius Wagner von Jauregg. *Wien.Klin.Wschr.*, 1947, 59: 130–132.

[64] Wagner-Jauregg. op.cit. ref 59.

[65] Wagner-Jauregg, op.cit. ref 59.

[66] Julius Wagner-Jauregg. Ueber die lanzinierenden Schmerzen der Tabetiker. *Wien.Klin.Wschr.*, 1924, 35: no. 40, 1046–48; Beziehungen zwischen Gelenks- und Nervenkrankheiten. *Wien.Med.Wschr.*, 1924, 74: no. 29, 1510–14; Ueber gastrische Krisen der Tabetiker und ihre Behandlung. *Wien.Klin.Wschr.*, 1926, 37: no. 38, 1093–95; Ueber tabische Optikusatrophie und deren Behandlung. *Z. Augenheilk.*, 1927, no. 3, 127–142.

[67] Wagner-Jauregg, op.cit. ref 12, p. 169.

[68] Julius Wagner-Jauregg. Einige Bemerkungen über Impfmalaria. *Wien.Klin.Wschr.*, 1927, 40: no. 1, 26–27.

[69] Julius Wagner-Jauregg. Einige Bemerkungen über die Impfmalaria. *Wien.Klin.Wschr.*, 1929, 42: no. 1, 1–2.

[70] R. Wethmar. Blutgruppen und Impf-Malaria. *Klin.Wschr.*, 1927, 6: 1947–48.

[71] Julius Wagner-Jauregg. Inwieweit besteht eine Gefährdung der Umgebung durch die therapeutische Malaria. *Wien.Klin.Wschr.*, 1933, 46: no. 23, 705–6.

[72] E. Martini. Grundsätzliches zur therapeutischen Malaria. *Dermatol.Wschr.*, 1932, no. 43, 1548–52.

[73] Julius Wagner-Jauregg. Ueber maximale Malariabehandlung der progressiven Paralyse. *Klin.Wschr.*, 1934, 13: no. 28, 1028.

[74] Julius Wagner-Jauregg. Die Behandlung der progressiven Paralyse mit Kurzwellen und Hochfrequenzströmen. *Wien.Med.Wschr.*, 1932, 82: no. 11, 328–32; 1934, 84: no. 1.

[75] Julius Wagner-Jauregg. Der Mechanismus der Wirkung der Infektions- und Fiebertherapie. *Klin.Wschr.*, 1935, 14: no. 14, 481–4.

[76] Julius Wagner-Jauregg. Drafts of letters to Paul de Kruif. Held at Institut für Geschichte der Medizin der Universität Wien.

[77] Paul de Kruif. *Men against Death*. London: Jonathan Cape, 1933.

[78] Julius Wagner-Jauregg. 'Infektions- und Fiebertherapie'. In *Handbuch der Neurologie*. Ed. O. Bumke und O. Foerster. Berlin: J. Springer, 1936.

[79] Julius Wagner-Jauregg. Fever therapy: its rationale in diseases of the nervous system. Cameron Lecture. *Edinburgh Med.J.*, 1936, 43: 1–12.

[80] Julius Wagner-Jauregg. Derzeitige Behandlung der progressiven

Paralyse. *Wien.Klin.Wschr.*, 1939, 52: no. 48, 1075–78.

[81] Julius Wagner-Jauregg. Letter to his son. Held at Institut für Geschichte der Medizin der Universität Wien.

[82] Wagner-Jauregg, op.cit. ref 19.

ELEVEN

LATER YEARS

After retirement from his chair and the directorship of the Clinic in 1928, Wagner-Jauregg continued with many of his activities and researches until a year or two before his death. He carried on with his private practice – he had many famous patients, including the well-known poet Josef Weinheber whom he treated for alcoholism (an exchange of letters has survived) and many actors. He continued with his work on the Senior Health Council, as there was no retiring age; he regularly attended the meetings of the Vienna Medical Society; and he maintained his research activities. Most of his papers on refinements and different aspects of his malaria therapy (discussed in Chapter 10) and on the campaign for goitre prophylaxis by the use of iodised salt (see Chapter 9) date from the 1920s and 1930s.

His earlier papers on general neurological and psychiatric problems were discussed in Chapters 2 and 3. There are, however, some papers on nervous and mental diseases of non-syphilitic origin that date from later years. He experimented with the use of fever therapy in the treatment of schizophrenics and manic-depressive patients and of multiple sclerosis, non-tubercular meningitis and diseases following encephalitis lethargica.[1] Looking back to his experiments with tuberculin in which good results had been obtained when a tubercular infection had been proved, he tried the method with schizophrenics with some success. He also suggested similar experiments with specific vaccines for mental patients also suffering from some infectious disease. As far as unspecific treatment was concerned, malaria or other fever therapy was tried in the case of manic-depressive patients and schizophrenics. However, the results

were not convincing. Wagner-Jauregg suggested that systematic controlled trials should be carried out on non-paralytic patients in
asylums to test the injection of infectious diseases or fever-causing
substances.

In the treatment of multiple sclerosis, which he believed to be
due to an infection, Wagner-Jauregg advocated the use of typhus
vaccine. He had noticed improvements in sufferers following an
infectious disease, just as he had in the case of mental diseases.
Tuberculin had no effect, but with staphylococcal vaccine there
were frequent remissions of symptoms. However, the best results he
obtained with typhus vaccine. Nevertheless, in a later paper he had
to admit that the experiments, which at first showed promising
results, did not lead to a complete and lasting remission of the
disease. In the treatment of non-tubercular meningitis, Wagner-
Jauregg recommended meningococcal sera or, if they were not available, staphylococcal vaccine. Another field of application for vaccine
treatment was septic infection. No improvements occurred when
he applied fever and infection therapy to the diseases following
encephalitis lethargica.

On one of these, Parkinsonism, he spoke in 1927 to a seminar
of physicians.[2] After the First World War encephalitis lethargica had
reached epidemic proportions and victims of this disease often began
to suffer from the consequences months or years after they had
recovered from the original infection. Apart from Parkinsonism, there
were movements of choreatic or athetotic character, also psychological consequences and manic symptoms. As far as treatment was
concerned, he discussed different methods and said that, although he
had not come across a cure, 'I am certainly not the man to preach
resignation; otherwise I would not have attained any success in
GPI.'

In a paper on organotherapy in neuroses and psychoses
Wagner-Jauregg,[3] after briefly reviewing the use of thyroid extract in
the malfunction of the thyroid, discussed the application of thyroid
therapy in cases of the disease of the pituitary gland. Different
surgical methods for extracting pituitary tumours had been carried
out, but mortality was high. It had, however, been found that
thyroid tablets could in some cases have a beneficial effect on vision.

Turning to the therapeutic use of sex gland substances,
Wagner-Jauregg said that, although dosages in thyroid therapy were
well established, knowledge of those in hormonal therapy was mini-
mal. Also, hormones were not usually given by mouth, the easier

method, but by subcutaneous or intramuscular injection. There was no doubt that the use of testicular substances inaugurated by C.E. Brown-Sequard (1817–94) in the treatment of impotence had good effect. He thought that the relation of mental and nervous disturbances, which occur during puberty, with internal secretion could justifiably be assumed. It was noticeable that the onset of Dementia praecox often fell into that period. Experience had shown that in cases of early hebephrenia treatment with thyroid extract and hormones could have a beneficial effect. In cases of young women suffering from a lack of sexual development and a mental illness it had been possible, by treatment with thyroid and ovarian preparations, to accelerate development and at the same time cure the psychosis. Similar treatment could cure ticks in young boys and girls which occurred during puberty.

Finally, Wagner-Jauregg turned to the method developed by Eugen Steinach (1864–1944) in 1920 involving the ligature of the vasa deferentia for rejuvenation. The method was hotly debated at four meetings of the Society for Psychiatry and Neurology in Vienna between January and April 1921, which Wagner-Jauregg noted in his diary – the only months for which entries survive. The procedure had already been carried out in America and also by himself on three youths whose physical and mental health had deteriorated to a dangerous extent as a result of excessive masturbation. Their health was considerably improved as a result of the operation. Wagner-Jauregg did not think that the consequent sterilisation was to be regretted as, in his opinion, persons with psychopathic constitutions should not procreate. On the success of Steinach's experiments for rejuvenation he was sceptical, but his experience in this respect was limited.

Two short articles dating from the late 1930s deal respectively with degenerative migraine and its treatment,[4] and sneezing.[5] The first distinguishes degenerative from normal migraine: the latter is of short duration, whereas the former, although the symptoms are similar, lasts much longer and does not respond to anti-neuralgic medication. It is often preceded by attacks of normal migraine which have occurred for years. Wagner-Jauregg called the article on sneezing a 'medical chat', it being a short historical note on the idea, going back to Homer, Hippocrates and Galen, that sneezing is beneficial. Powders to cause sneezing were listed in old pharmacopoeias, and snuff tobacco was popular after Francois II used it to treat headache. He wondered whether Hippocrates's idea about the relation between nose and brain could be sustained. Hydrorhoea nasalis, caused by brain tumours, and hydrocephalus, in which liquor pressure was increased, could be alleviated by means which produced sneezing.

Among Wagner-Jauregg's papers there is a manuscript on 'Aconite for trigeminal neuralgia', of which no published version has been found.[6] In it he described a method he had used for forty years in treating trigeminal neuralgia, originally suggested by Seguin[7] who had emphasised that the treatment with aconite required the physician to combine caution with courage. Caution was needed because of the toxicity of aconite and the impossibility of fixing a definite dose because of the difference in patients' sensitivity. Courage was required to increase the dosage so as to achieve a satisfactory therapeutic effect. The treatment was not intended to replace surgery, but could be used post-operatively and repeated at will.

THE CRAZE FOR PSYCHICAL EXPERIMENTS

After the end of the First World War and in the early 1920s, Wagner-Jauregg became very concerned about the craze (he called it an epidemic) for public shows of hypnotism and psychical phenomena. Already in an address to the Vienna Medical Society in June 1919[8] on 'Suggestion, Hypnotism and Telepathy' he voiced his criticism of these public shows and emphasised their danger. He followed H. Bernheim (1840–1919) in believing that the hypnotic state could only come about by way of suggestion; on the other hand, suggestibility was increased by hypnosis. Suggestion could be effective without hypnosis, through so-called 'awake hypnosis' and hypnotic suggestion. The significance of the latter could not be overestimated, particularly in criminal cases. Certain individuals through their strong personality could exert so much influence on one or a group of persons that they had no resistance and accepted all their orders obediently. If this state lasted for any length of time, they became compliant and mentally enslaved. Wagner-Jauregg spoke of the danger of post-hypnotic suggestion which could lead to a misuse of hypnosis for criminal purposes. Speaking of experiments carried out daily by professional and amateur hypnotists, to the astonishment of those present at public shows and also in private circles, it was difficult to be sure whether the medium was really in a hypnotic state or was only play-acting.

As far as telepathy was concerned, what was being demonstrated in Vienna was not telepathy but thought-reading. Wagner-Jauregg did not dispute the possibility of perceiving the thoughts of other persons, although they were not communicated verbally or in writing, but he was very sceptical as to the possibility of genuine telepathic communication on the strength of the available evidence.

Some documents dating back to January/July 1924[9] make it clear that, although Wagner-Jauregg was ready to examine parapsychic phenomena, he soon became very much opposed not only to public shows, but also to the setting up of institutions investigating these. According to a draft dated January 1924, an interdisciplinary Committee was formed, consisting of a number of members of the Professorial Board including M. Schlick (1882–1936), Professor of Philosophy, K. Bühler (1879–1963), Professor of Psychology, A. Durig (b. 1872), Professor of Physiology, F. Ehrenhaft (1879–1952), Professor of Physics, and Wagner-Jauregg who seems to have acted as Chairman. The draft of a request for a meeting with two mediums, Rudi and Willy Schneider, addressed to the persons under whose protection they were kept, was signed by him. There is also the draft of a note to the Director of an Institute (presumably H. Thirring, the Director of the Institute of Physics, since the documents include several letters by him on the subject), to allow members of the Committee to observe the experiments carried out. A letter from H. Thirring, dated 22 April 1924, states that experiments with one of the two mediums had taken place on 15 April but the results were negative. It was planned to continue the experiments at the Institute, and as soon as the mediums had become acclimatised to the surroundings, and provided that any psychic phenomena occurred, the Committee would be asked to attend. There are two further letters from H. Thirring: in the first, dated 23 June, Thirring says that he would like to report to the Committee on the results of the experiments and he suggested a date for the visit. In the other, dated 9 July, Thirring expresses his regrets at Professor Durig's intention to resign from the Committee and requests Wagner-Jauregg to call a meeting of the Committee so that those who had taken part in the experiments would have an opportunity to exchange views with the remaining Committee members. A letter dated 9 July, signed by Wagner-Jauregg and addressed to an 'Esteemed Colleague' (presumably H. Thirring), states that 'The direction which the experiments planned by the Committee for the investigation of occult phenomena has taken causes me to resign from the Committee. Professor Durig has joined me in this step.'

Four reports prepared at the request of the Senior Health Council in the course of 1924[10] leave no doubt as to Wagner-Jauregg's attitude in these matters. The first concerned an appeal by a general practitioner against the refusal by the provincial health office for permission to organise lectures on the nature of suggestion, combined with demonstrations of the phenomenon. Wagner-Jauregg argued forcibly against allowing the appeal. He was particularly concerned with the damage to health both of the mediums and those attending shows of this kind. He was in favour of a general prohibition of public shows of experiments with hypnosis and suggestion, not only by laymen but also by physicians. There was no objection to theoretical lectures on the subject and no need to stop physicians from using hypnosis for curative purposes.

The second report related to the establishment of a 'Vienna Metapsychological Institute' as a private research institute for the exploration and promotion of metapsychology, parapsychology or parapsychophysics (a new special science) by two persons, one of whom was a doctor of medicine. The aim of the institute was to organise lectures with slides, experiments in the field of clairvoyance and in the field of physical phenomena, such as levitation, telekinesis, and phenomena of materialization. The Vienna magistrates requested the Ministry for Social Welfare for guidance regarding the Institute and this was passed on to the Senior Health Council which in turn asked Wagner-Jauregg to report. Wagner-Jauregg contended that, whatever attitude one took towards the tendencies to acquire knowledge beyond the limits set by time and space and physical conditions, the experience of psychiatric clinics showed that experiments to produce different occult phenomena could lead to health hazards for those taking part. He recommended that the performance of occult experiments open to the general public and their announcement should be prohibited; no note should be taken of the establishment of the Vienna Metapsychological Institute; and an eye should be kept on abuses in this field.

The third report also concerned the setting up of an institute for the systematic and unprejudiced research into and education in psychical phenomena according to academic principles, called the 'Vienna Psychical Institute'. To achieve these goals it was proposed to carry out pertinent experiments, to organise regular popular scientific lectures on all problems of occultism and to establish a library, a collection of technical aids and an institute journal. The Vienna Police authorities proposed to prohibit the setting up of the Institute because in Austria experiments in spiritism, occultism and hypnosis were forbidden by law. Furthermore, the provincial government had ruled that public performances of waking suggestion and experiments on members of the public could damage the health of those involved in them. Consequently, the competent Magistrate ruled that the setting up of the Institute was against the law, whereupon the person who made the proposal appealed and Wagner-Jauregg was asked for his report. In this he repeated the conclusions he had arrived at in the previous case and argued against the appeal being allowed.

During the following year another application for the approval of the establishment of a 'Society for Research into Mediums' was turned down by the Vienna Magistrate, again because of possible health hazards. The proposers of the application appealed and the Office of Public Health requested a report from the Senior Health Council which Wagner-Jauregg was asked to submit. In this he referred to his reports on the three cases mentioned above and recommended that the appeal should be rejected for the same reasons. However, he even went further in suggesting that the Office of Public Health should issue a general prohibition of the promotion of supernatural problems through the activities of societies which had great propagandist influence.[11]

HEREDITY AND EUGENICS

Already in his first Inaugural Lecture upon appointment to the Chair of Psychiatry at the University of Vienna in 1893, Wagner-Jauregg discussed the role of heredity in the aetiology of mental diseases.[12] Heredity not only gave rise to a latent disposition towards these, but also to distinct characteristics in the descendants which distinguished them from the mass of the healthy population. Clearly much influenced by Morel's theory of degeneration and Lombroso's ideas, Wagner-Jauregg described to his students the mental and physical characteristics of degenerate individuals, which they were likely to encounter in their practice. Although the principal inherited mental disorders concerned feelings and affects, degenerate persons also showed certain physical characteristics, mostly of an anatomical but also of a functional nature, indicating defects of internal organisation. Few of them played an important role in social life, but some had outstanding talents and were to be found at the top of social, political, religious and aesthetic movements. However, the majority ended up in lunatic asylums or prisons, or else became anarchists and were responsible for such horrors as the Paris Commune.

Leaving aside the question of hereditary degeneration, Wagner-Jauregg dealt with the nature of crime and distinguished between occasional and born criminals. In this connection, he referred to Lombroso's hypothesis that the characteristics of the born criminal may essentially be interpreted as atavisms, i.e. as a reversal to an earlier state of development. Lombroso had mentioned two characteristics which tended to occur in criminals, rather than in ordinary, healthy individuals: the medial occipital cavity (Forsa occiputalis) is found in a far smaller percentage of healthy people than in criminals and there are far fewer left-handed among the healthy. There was also a noticeable predilection of criminals for tattooing!

Wagner-Jauregg, unlike Lombroso, considered criminal nature or moral insanity to be a mental illness. He thought of criminals as sick people. They tended to epilepsy and mental derangement, but it was difficult to decide how much was due to their constitution and what part was played by external influences, such as social factors, education and environment.

In connection with the ideas put forward in this lecture, Wagner-Jauregg suggested to one of his assistants, A. Pilcz, that he make some comparisons between degenerates and paralytics. In the article which Pilcz[13] published as the result of his researches, he concluded that in GPI heredity did not play a considerable part and that insanity occurred seldom in the prehistory of paralytics. He quoted a number of authors who maintained that there was no GPI without syphilitic infection. Pilcz's paper was severely criticised by P. Naecke (1851–1913),[14] who had previously written on the subject.[15] Remembering his polemics with Moebius (*see* Chapter 3), Wagner-Jauregg replied on Pilcz's behalf as he, of course, had much greater authority. His paper 'On the constitution of paralytics' was published in 1900.[16] The argument turned largely on the statistical methods used by Naecke and Pilcz. The main conclusions reached by Pilcz and supported by Wagner-Jauregg was that heredity did not play as great a part in paralytics as in other insane patients. Another point of contention seems to have been the phenomenon of tattooing which Pilcz considered a sign of degeneration, whereas Naecke did not attribute any significance to it.

The main theme of Wagner-Jauregg's second Inaugural Lecture,[17] delivered on the occasion of his assuming the direction of the

Second Psychiatric Clinic in 1902, was that heredity was the most important factor in all mental diseases. After some references to the work of his predecessors at the Second Clinic, Meynert and Krafft-Ebing, he spoke of the importance of statistical methods in the investigation of heredity in mental disease. He based his remarks on the researches carried out by Jenny Koller under the direction of Forel at Zürich, which he examined critically. It was not easy to prove that a mental disease could be inherited, only the disposition to the disease. The contemporary theory of heredity presumed a unity of psychopathic disposition, whereas mental disease took many forms. Koller's study led to the conclusion that mental disease occurred more often in a family with bad mental health than in a healthy family, but Wagner-Jauregg wanted more evidence and urged the reform of the prevailing theory of heredity.

From further statistical results compiled by the Zürich Psychiatric Clinic,[18] which were based on a far greater number of individuals, Wagner-Jauregg concluded that the figures proved that adverse heredity was not the only, nor even the decisive cause of mental illness. Again he stressed that mental illness itself could not be inherited, only a disposition or immunity to it. A surprising result of the statistics was that families in whom nervous diseases occurred tended to show some degree of immunity to mental disturbance. Wagner-Jauregg emphasised the rare occurrence of GPI among degenerates and psychopaths; on the other hand, epilepsy and certain other mental diseases were often found among them.

Wagner-Jauregg reverted to the subject of the rôle of heredity in nervous and mental diseases many years later, in 1928,[19] when Mendel's theories* had become widely known and had given rise to a major turning point in biology. He claimed that Mendel's laws were based on a large number of individuals who were under the same environmental influences, and did not apply to the family; also in biology the theory was amenable to experiment, whereas in pathology it was not possible to provide proof experimentally. Moreover, external influences were likely to modify the disposition to disease.

As regards GPI, it was not possible to determine whether heredity, either in the disposition or immunity to the disease, played a rôle because it only occurred after a syphilitic infection. Nervous

---

* J.G. Mendel (1822–84).

diseases, being familial, were more likely to elucidate the principles of heredity. Wagner-Jauregg queried whether heredity alone was sufficient to cause them or whether external influences were needed for the disease to appear.

In the case of Huntington's chorea,* which was caused by a dominant gene, heredity was direct from parents to children, and it was not possible for a generation to be passed over. The situation regarding the disease was not as simple as in Mendel's experiments with peas. It had been shown that one or other of the characteristic symptoms, e.g. choreatic muscular disquiet, psychological disturbances, and progressive course, did not occur and that it was even possible that there was no chorea. Such differences were even observed in members of the same family. Wagner-Jauregg queried how so many differing symptoms could result from an hereditary disposition.

This many-sided symptomology was also present in the familial nervous disease which was characterised by Friedreich's ataxia[†] at one end and Marie's hereditary cerebellar ataxia[‡] at the other, which showed quite different symptoms. It had been established that Marie's ataxia was caused by a dominant gene, whereas Friedreich's was a consequence of recessive heredity. How was it possible then, Wagner-Jauregg wondered, that these two diseases occurred in the same family?

It was found in biological experiments that dominance and recessivity were not absolute quantities but may be present in all possible proportions and that hereditary factors must therefore be considered not only qualitatively, but also quantitatively. It was therefore possible for one and the same disease to be caused by a dominant gene in one family and by a recessive one in another. Moreover, environmental influences might be at work.

Some authorities had emphasised that in order to form a proper judgment on the course of congenital diseases, it was necessary to consider what were called 'formes frustes', healthy persons who nevertheless showed some mild symptoms of the disease. Discussing the so-called correlation of hereditary traits, that is the regular occurrence of two hereditary characteristics in one individual, Wagner-

---

* G.S. Huntington (1850–1916).
[†] Nikolaus Friedreich (1826–82).
[‡] Pierre Marie (1853–1940).

Jauregg referred to the combination of myotonic muscular dystrophy and cataracts.

The endocrine system and its functions were affected by heredity, as for example in diabetes and Basedow's disease. Many authors believed that it played a considerable rôle in schizophrenia and even in manic-depressive psychosis. On the other hand, the endocrine system was greatly influenced by environmental factors, as in goitre.

Reverting to a discussion of congenital nervous diseases, Wagner-Jauregg considered muscular dystrophy and its symptoms in the light of the contemporary literature. One remarkable fact was the frequent occurrence of sporadic cases in which no familial heredity could be proved. As it was supposed to follow a dominant course, this presented a difficulty. Whether it was due to a mutation was questionable.

In the second part of this lengthy paper, Wagner-Jauregg discussed the progress of the theory of heredity as applied to mental diseases. These, following Kraepelin, he considered in two groups, namely manic-depressive psychoses and schizophrenia, but he added epilepsy as a third. The study of heredity had confirmed the correctness of Kraepelin's conception of manic-depressive disease because it was found that in one and the same family both manic and melancholic states occurred, either separately or in a cyclic and periodic fashion. Wagner-Jauregg asked himself how two such different syndromes could alternate not only in a family, but in one individual, and what was it that was inherited. He concluded that two factors were involved: an abnormally high instability and a periodic factor that was often found in the animal and plant world but not usually in man. He ventured the hypothesis that in some human families periodicity might have been retained as a hereditary feature. However, he thought that environmental influences determined the occurrence at different ages and different times in an individual with a manic-depressive disposition.

The problems posed by schizophrenia were more difficult for two reasons: first, it was doubtful whether schizophrenia represented one disease or several pathological processes which were only loosely connected by their symptoms. Secondly, the hereditary factor was not nearly so distinctive as in manic-depressive illness. Wagner-Jauregg quoted some authorities who believed that schizophrenia was due to a combination of two different hereditary traits which separately did not lead to the disease. He questioned whether one of these might not be hereditary, but environmental or due to damage to the foetus. This would explain why children of those suffering from schizophrenia seldom had the disease.

Speaking of the two main groups of psychoses, it seemed that, although manic-depressive psychoses had been observed in parents with children suffering from schizophrenia, the opposite was hardly ever the case. In families in which both groups of diseases occurred there were many individuals who, although not mentally ill, showed characteristics of one or the other group, and these were referred to as cycloid and schizoid personalities. They were correlated with body-build by Kretschmer* who distinguished between pyknic, asthenic and athletic build, finding that cycloid personalities were almost always of the pyknic build, whereas the schizoid type usually belonged to the other two body-builds.

As far as epilepsy was concerned, Wagner-Jauregg thought that environmental factors played a dominant rôle and that heredity was a minor factor.

The article concludes with a short discussion of the problem of marriage between relatives. Wagner-Jauregg thought that the danger that a recessive disposition to an illness may be latent in a family, and only appear in their offspring, could not be excluded, and he warned of marriages between closely related people. Finally, he stressed that although heredity must not be neglected, disease was a product of two factors, heredity and environment.

A year later, in a lecture to the Austrian Society for Improving the Nation and for Heredity,[20] Wagner-Jauregg repeated the main arguments put forward in the lengthy article published in 1928, but it is clear that the interest of the lecture, as might be expected in view of the audience, was their impact on eugenics, particularly on marriage counselling. The lecture concludes with a short discussion of heredity in groups of men with criminal tendencies. The danger of inheriting criminal and asocial dispositions was increased by the fact that the spouses of such individuals often brought with them a similar disposition since 'birds of a feather flock together'.

Wagner-Jauregg became increasingly concerned with problems of eugenics and was elected President of the Society to whom the lecture was addressed. In an article in 1931[21] he outlined the aim of eugenics which was to exclude, as far as possible, persons with adverse hereditary traits from procreation, and to encourage those

---

*Ernst Kretschmer (1888–1964).

with favourable traits. However, the former policy would reduce population growth and thus diminish the standing of the country among other states. Therefore, steps in this direction had to be considered carefully. In the first instance, those with hereditary mental defects and those with criminal tendencies should be prevented from procreation, but the difficulty was how to achieve this goal. The two suggestions Wagner-Jauregg put forward were propaganda among the people and marriage counselling. However, centres established for this purpose had reported poor attendance and it was clear that interest in eugenics had not been aroused.

With regard to measures preventing the mentally ill and those with criminal tendencies from procreating, according to the Austrian interdiction order of 1916, those who were under guardianship were allowed to marry if the Court gave its consent. In discussions on the subject the problem of sterilisation was in the forefront. In the United States vasectomies for eugenic purposes had been carried out since 1899, five States providing for voluntary sterilisation, seven for voluntary and compulsory, and seven for compulsory only. Switzerland followed suit, and other countries introduced laws regulating sterilisation. In Germany and Austria the Eugenics Societies had sent proposals to Parliament for legalising sterilisation for eugenic purposes.

Dealing with the second task of eugenics, Wagner-Jauregg believed that it was the higher social classes that ought to be encouraged to have larger families. They gave a bad example to the rest by not having enough offspring. Wagner-Jauregg had made a short statistical study concerning the families of thirty-four men who passed the final examination at his school the year he did, and found that they had had only thirty-four children – that is, half the total needed to maintain their number. He pleaded for members to encourage an interest in eugenics in the country and become members of the Eugenics Society.

In the year in which this article appeared Wagner-Jauregg was asked by Marianne Hainisch (1839–1936), an eminent fighter for women's rights, to address a meeting of women at which the Papal Encyclical of December 1930, *Casti connubii*, on Christian marriage, was to be discussed. The original of his reply, which is in the Library of the City and Province of Vienna (Wiener Stadt- und Landesbibliothek), gives his reasons for declining the invitation after serious consideration. The main reason he gave was that, even if he stressed that the opinions expressed were his own, it might be thought that as he was the President of the Eugenics Society he was voicing the Society's opinions. Since its members held very different views and the Society was apolitical, it would give offence to some if he engaged in polemics on the Encyclical. Moreover, he did not think it opportune for persons who shared his views to comment officially on the Papal announcements. This would cause controversy and nothing would be gained by it. Many who held no definite views might be driven into opposition, and this would have the opposite effect of what he was hoping to achieve. It must be remembered that many Austrian legislative ordinances and legal decisions were not in agreement with the orders contained in the Encyclical. A heated polemic on it might endanger progress, for example on legislation regarding marriage and in other fields where some progress had already been made. 'I believe', Wagner-Jauregg wrote, 'that we should approach the legislative authorities without discussing the Encyclical which did not contain new orders, but only repeated old ones.' No meetings or speeches would induce the Curia to change its point of view, but established facts had occasionally done that in the past. He was surprised to see that the Encyclical allowed sterilisation under very stringent conditions.

In an article a few years later,[22] in which he repeated most of the arguments put forward in the 1931 paper, he referred to the Encyclical, which in principle objected to eugenic sterilisation, except in the case of criminals. Wagner-Jauregg was pessimistic regarding voluntary marriage counselling, and suggested that prospective spouses should by law be made to produce certificates to show that they were fit to marry. He advocated a prohibition on the marriage of blood relations and economic help for couples who were likely to produce healthy offspring. It was unfortunate that the healthier classes produced fewer children, but it was difficult to discriminate in this area. Finally, Wagner-Jauregg advocated the spread of eugenic knowledge in schools and the encouragement of pupils to study their family histories.

Wagner-Jauregg's ideas on heredity and eugenics permeate a book *On the human life span*,[23] the manuscript of which was found on his desk when he died and published by his son. It is a short semi-popular work in which he discusses the life span of different species, including plants and animals, and the life span of the individual, based mainly on German statistics. The theory of heredity forms the central part of the book. In it he deals with congenital diseases in man and hereditary aspects of the life span of the individual, and in later chapters with ageing and longevity, the effect of maturity of the parents on the life span of the children, and marriages between individuals belonging to the same family. In the last chapter he questions whether life can be lengthened by human activity. The time-interval between conception and death was the field of activity of the physician and above all the social hygienist. The production of a most favourable genotype was the task of the physician and the legislator as racial hygienist. The elimination of the worst mutations causing congenital diseases had been initiated by the German race protection laws. However, they could not prevent the appearance of new mutations. Wagner-Jauregg did not think that X-rays had a noticeable effect, but wondered whether excessive exposure to sunlight might. Measures should be taken to avoid alcohol, nicotine, and drugs before the period of childbearing.

His final question was: 'Is the promotion of longevity desirable?' He took the view that it was not for the general good for there to be a large number of individuals nearing the maximum life span, since they became a charge on the younger members of the population and often disagreed with contemporary ideas and principles. However, since increased vitality and fertility were desirable, it would be necessary to resign oneself to greater longevity.

REFERENCES

[1] Julius Wagner-Jauregg. Vakzinetherapie der Nervenkrankheiten. *Wien.Med.Wschr.*, 1922, 72: no. 1, 3; Fieber- und Infektions-therapie von Nerven- und Geisteskrankheiten. Ibid. 1930, 80: no. 20, 651–654; Ueber spezifische und Unspecifische Behandlung von Geisteskrankheiten. *Deut.Nervenheilk.*, 1931, 117/119: 672 et seq.

[2] Julius Wagner-Jauregg. Ueber Parkinsonismus. *Wien.Klin.Wschr.*, 1927, 40: no. 48, 1529–32.

[3] Julius Wagner-Jauregg. Organotherapie bei Neurosen und Psychosen. *Wien.Klin.Wschr.*, 1923, 36: 1–4.

[4] Julius Wagner-Jauregg. Ueber ausgeartete Migräne und ihre Behandlung. *Wien.Med.Wschr.*, 1935, 85: no. 1, 1–2.

[5] Julius Wagner-Jauregg. Ueber das Niesen. *Wien.Med.Wschr.*, 1936, 86: no. 1, 9–12.

[6] Julius Wagner-Jauregg. MS. held at Institut für Geschichte der Medizin der Universität Wien.

7 E. Seguin. Report on aconitia in Trigeminal Neuralgia. *New York Medical Journal*, 1878, 28: 621–628.

8 Julius Wagner-Jauregg. Ueber Suggestion, Hypnose und Telepathie. *Wien.Med.Wschr.*, 1919, 69: no. 27, 1333–1338: no. 28, 1384–90.

9 Correspondence held at Institut für Geschichte der Medizin der Universität Wien.

10 Julius Wagner-Jauregg. Drei Gutachten des Obersten Sanitätsrates, betreffend Demonstrationsvorträge auf dem Gebiete des Hypnotismus, der 'Metapsychologie' und der 'Parapsychologie'. *Wien.Klin.Wschr.*, 1925, 38: no. 43, 1163–67.

11 Julius Wagner-Jauregg. Bildung des Vereines 'Gesellschaft für Medienforschung'; Untersagung. *Mitteilungen des Volksgesundheitsamtes*, July 1925, no. 7, 298–299.

12 Julius Wagner-Jauregg. Antrittsvorlesung an der psychiatrischen Klinik in der Landesirrenanstalt. *Wien.Klin.Wschr.*, 1893, 6: no. 47, 848–852.

13 A. Pilcz. Ueber Beziehungen zwischen Paralyse und Degeneration. *Monatsschr.Psychiat.Neurol.*, 1899, 6: 1–14.

14 P. Naecke. Dementia paralytica und Degeneration. *Neurol. Centralbl.*, 1899, 18: no. 24, 1121–30.

15 P. Naecke. Die sogenannten äusseren Degenerationszeichen bei der progressiven Paralyse der Männer. *Allg.Z.Psychiat.*, 1898, 55: 557–693.

16 Julius Wagner-Jauregg. Zur Veranlagung der Paralytiker. *Monatsschr.Psychiat.Neurol.*, 1900, 8: no. 5, 325–336.

17 Julius Wagner-Jauregg. Ueber erbliche Belastung. *Wien.Klin. Wschr.*, 1906, 19: no. 1, 1–6.

18 Julius Wagner-Jauregg. Einiges über erbliche Belastung. *Wien. Klin.Wschr.*, 1906, 19: no. 1, 1–6.

19 Julius Wagner-Jauregg. Ueber Erblichkeit in der Pathologie. *Wien.Klin.Wschr.*, 1928, 41: no. 16, 545–549; no. 17, 595–598.

20 Julius Wagner-Jauregg. Die erbliche Anlage zu Geistesstörungen. *Wien.Klin.Wschr.*, 1929, 42: no. 28, 925–927; no. 29, 961–963.

21 Julius Wagner-Jauregg. Ueber Eugenik. *Wien.Klin.Wschr.*, 1931, 44: no. 1, 1–6.

22 Julius Wagner-Jauregg. Zeitgemässe Eugenik. *Wien.Klin.Wschr.*, 1935, 48: no. 1, 1–2.

23 Julius Wagner-Jauregg. *Ueber die menschliche Lebensdauer.* Eine populär-wissenschaftliche Darstellung. Innsbruck: Deutscher Alpenverlag, 1941.

TWELVE

WAGNER-JAUREGG – THE FINAL CHAPTER

Wagner-Jauregg's career was a success story from the time he joined the First Psychiatric Clinic as an assistant, to his attainment of the renowned position of Director of the Second Psychiatric Clinic at the General Hospital, and his appointment to the Professorial Board and to the Senior Health Council. His marriage to Balbine Frumkin, whom he thought to have cured of her morphine addiction, seems to have been extremely unhappy. In his *Memoirs* Wagner-Jauregg never mentions anything relating to his personal affairs and few letters survive touching on any such matters. What we know is based on his son's autobiography, some reminiscences by his son and the sons of his stepdaughter, Melanie, and a few documents found among his archives. According to Melanie's sons, Balbine had a relapse, disrupted his private practice and created havoc in his household. A note, recently discovered among Wagner-Jauregg's papers, signed by Balbine and dated September 1898, makes sad reading. It states 'I confirm herewith that my husband, at my urgent and repeated entreaties, has declared himself willing to continue living with me only under certain conditions agreed by us.' This does not suggest a happy marriage, although a daughter was born in July 1900. Nevertheless, the marriage became so unhappy that a separation was agreed upon. A document, which survives, dated November 1903, contains the legal arrangements for the custody of the child. Already during that year Wagner-Jauregg described himself as 'geschieden' (separated or divorced). However, no legal divorce was possible according to the law then valid in Austria. After the break-up of their marriage, Balbine moved to an apartment in one of the inner suburbs where she lived with their daughter Julie, but her elder daughter, Melanie, Wagner-Jauregg's stepdaughter, was brought up in her step-father's household in the large apartment in the centre of the city where he resided from 1892 until his death in 1940.

By 1902 his marriage must have broken down irretrievably. During that year he became acquainted with a young woman, Anna Koch, who acted as a companion and nurse to depressed patients. She had had a very sad childhood, having lost her mother at an early age. She was brought up first by a stepmother who was rather unkind and afterwards in an orphanage. From the age of fourteen she had to fend for herself. She was 22 when she met Wagner-Jauregg, who was then 45, and a son was born to them in 1903, named Theodor as a 'gift of God' and also in memory of Julius's friend and colleague, Theodor Escherich. In his biography Theodor, who later became a distinguished pharmaceutical chemist, says 'As my father had no male descendant and did not want his name to die out, he decided to attempt once again to have a family.' Of course, since Wagner-Jauregg's first marriage could not be dissolved, Theodor remained illegitimate, bearing his mother's name, Koch, until Wagner-Jauregg was able to marry his mother after the death of his first wife in 1924. Theodor writes that his father married his mother when he realized that his son was a very good student. Whether Wagner-Jauregg made this statement with his tongue in cheek is not known, but it is a fact that he still continued to live on his own after the marriage.

In his earliest childhood, Theodor was led to believe that his father was an uncle. He describes a holiday trip to the Adriatic with his mother and father when a fellow traveller asked where his father was. He was puzzled when his reply that he had no father but that his uncle was very good to him caused some merriment. Wagner-Jauregg visited his son and his son's mother for a few hours every second or third day. Only when the son was grown up did they return his visits. Theodor and his mother lived with one servant in one of the outer suburbs of Vienna in an apartment typical of this lower-middle-class district. When it was time for Theodor to leave the elementary school and go on to high school, they moved to a more prosperous neighbourhood in one of the inner suburbs. Often on Sundays Wagner-Jauregg took his son on walks into the Vienna woods or on an outing into the hills further away. Being a good botanist, he imparted his knowledge to his son, and in later years medical colleagues joined these excursions, arousing Theodor's interest in medical problems. Although they did not share a home, father, mother and son went quite often on holiday together. It is clear from Theodor Wagner-Jauregg's autobiography that he held his father in great respect and that in turn Wagner-Jauregg was very proud of his son's scientific achievements – a fact confirmed by the few letters from father to son that have survived. Theodor writes that, although in his adult life he met many important persons, he admired none more than his father, whose personality was so striking and impressive.

Wagner-Jauregg seems to have been very attached both to his daughter Julie and his step-daughter Mela. Julie in later years became a well-known traveller and for six years explored the French Sahara. At the invitation of the Geographical Society of Vienna she gave two illustrated lectures on 'The Sahara and its inhabitants' and on 'The Tuareg Romantics of the Sahara' in October 1928 and received well-earned applause. In one of the reminiscences of Wagner-Jauregg it is told that her father was against her accepting the invitation, but when the lectures were well-received he said to a friend of his daughter, 'I may perhaps become famous through my daughter'. Among the few diary entries that have been preserved from the last month of his life, he notes the arrival of some photographs of his daughter Julie.

There is not much doubt about his attachment to his step-daughter Mela who must at some time or another have acted as his secretary. There are several notes in the draft letters among his archives, 'Mela. Please let me have one copy.'; 'Mela. Please check my translation.' Mela married Max Ungethüm and they had two sons who were devoted to their 'Grandpapa'. The name Ungethüm occurs in many notes and there are several references to meetings and outings with them. In a postcard dated 9 August 1936, now in the Archives of the City and Province of Vienna (Wiener Stadt-und Landesarchiv), addressed to a Dr Jenny Rieder and written from a Restaurant where, as he said, he was drowning his worries in a green 'Silvaner' (an Austrian white wine), he wrote how worried he was about Mela whom he found to be suffering from an abdominal tumour which he feared might be malignant, and which would probably necessitate an operation.* This would be the end of his summer holidays.

---

* Mela Ungethüm did not die until January 1971.

According to his assistant Stransky, Wagner-Jauregg had few close friends. He thought that the only one of his colleagues who deserved that description was Constantin von Economo (1876–1931) with whose widow he became joint author of his biography. In later years a Dr John became a friend and his name appears in the late diary entries. There are also drafts of correspondence with Adolf Lorenz, the famous orthopaedic surgeon, who had been a fellow student and remained a friend for life.

WAGNER-JAUREGG'S POLITICAL VIEWS

As might be expected, in politics Wagner-Jauregg was very conservative and a German nationalist. Like many people of his generation he believed that since Austria's culture was essentially Germanic, despite its multi-national structure during the days of the Empire, it should be part of Germany. He supported the student fraternities that were in favour of the *Anschluss* and gave them financial support. As to his attitude to Jews there are different opinions. His son, replying to a letter, wrote 'there is no question of my father being antisemitic, otherwise his clinical assistants and colleagues would not have been mainly Jews.' On the other hand, his assistant Stransky, himself of Jewish origin and a great admirer of his teacher, told a different story in his autobiography and there are a few remarks in Wagner-Jauregg's own *Memoirs* that suggest that he was not fond of Jews generally, although he was always just to his Jewish assistants and students, whom he valued as men and scientists and whom he helped when it was in his power. He also acknowledged his debt to his Jewish teachers. He disliked Jewish jokes for which he had no understanding. Although very witty, he took himself very seriously and lacked what might be called the English type of humour.

There is a short passage in the autobiography of Arthur Schnitzler (1862–1931), the well-known Austrian writer, which must refer to Wagner-Jauregg. It says 'At the Gymnasium (high school) there were few traces of antisemitism. Among those – professors now – Wagnerianer, German nationalist, pronounces Jewish first names in a mocking fashion, but commits no injustices, marries a Jewess.'

His attitude to Jews is typical of that of many Austrians, such as Karl Lueger, the mayor of Vienna, whose party was extremely antisemitic, and who said 'I decide who is a Jew'. After all Wagner-Jauregg married a Jewess, but it is doubtful whether the unhappiness

198

of the marriage caused his anti-Jewish feelings. Also his devotion to his stepdaughter, who was of Jewish origin, speaks against this. He was not pleased when many young Jewish doctors joined his Clinic, not only because of his general dislike of Jews, but because they were likely to give him more trouble than the gentiles since they encountered more difficulties in their careers.

There is documentary evidence that in his later years Wagner-Jauregg joined the Nazi party, although his son wrote that he did not know whether this was so. At the Memorial Meeting of the newly formed Vienna Medical Society (replacing the old Society which admitted Jews), ten days after Wagner-Jauregg's death, the 'Gauamtsleiter' of the Office of Public Health (a Nazi official) spoke of Wagner-Jauregg's public approval of Hitler's actions and of national socialist ideas. He said that he was the first to sign the roll of members of the new medical society already planned in 1937 (a year before the Anschluss) and that he accepted national socialist ideas with enthusiasm.

Although one might query the enthusiasm, the facts are incontrovertible. However, Wagner-Jauregg's son believed that his father had hoped that Hitler would settle the injustices of the Versailles treaty peacefully and was very disappointed in Hitler's behaviour after his election as Chancellor. Erwin Stengel (1902–73), who emigrated to England after the Anschluss and became Professor of Psychiatry at Sheffield, was told by Wagner-Jauregg that there was no need to emigrate because 'the situation would soon settle down.' Stransky wrote that, although Wagner-Jauregg was in favour of German nationalism and at first supported National Socialism, when he saw how things were developing he did not withhold his criticism, particularly of the idea of disposing of the mentally ill and feeble, and also of other Nazi measures. Stransky relates how, after Wagner-Jauregg's cremation which he attended, he spoke to Professor L. Arzt (b. 1883) who had supported the Dollfuss and Schuschnigg regimes and was imprisoned by the Nazis for a short time. Professor Arzt told him that immediately after his release he was visited by Wagner-Jauregg, with whom he had not been on particularly good terms, who wanted to show his opposition to Hitler's brutality. There is also the testimony of M. Gerstmann, the widow of one of Wagner-Jauregg's assistants who had to emigrate to the United States: she writes 'When Austria succumbed to the Nazis, Wagner-Jauregg was one of the very few whose integrity was unflinching.' During those months, although over 80 years old, he came daily to the Institution where her husband was Director, to register patients who were being persecuted either for political or religious reasons, thereby protecting them and her husband from an accusation of hiding persons wanted by the Gestapo.

WAGNER-JAUREGG'S LIFE-STYLE

Wagner-Jauregg's life-style was that of a well-to-do professional man. Living in a large apartment near the centre of the city in the district where most medical men had their practices, he was looked after by two servants, a parlour-maid and a cook. He was not fond of parties or official gatherings and avoided large conferences whenever possible, preferring to entertain colleagues and family to luncheon or dinner at his home. His cook was well known for her delicious cooking. Sometimes colleagues even called on him at breakfast-time on their way to the hospital.

Some diary entries for January to April 1921, which Professor Theodor Wagner-Jauregg kindly placed at the author's disposal, illustrate his father's daily activities. The first entry is for New Year's Eve, 1920, when there must have been a small party. Apart from his daughter Julie five other names are mentioned and the only entry under Saturday, 1 January is 'Hangover'. Nevertheless on the following Sunday, the sun was shining and he was off with his daughter and his stepdaughter's husband on an excursion to the 'Eisernes Tor' (the Iron Gate), a mountain some twenty miles from Vienna, which seems to have been a favourite place of his. The diary continues with notes on meetings in his apartment, lectures and attendances at different professional meetings, dinner engagements, and items of general interest such as a postal strike, a telephone strike and the increase in the value of the Austrian currency. Most Sundays he is out walking to some place in the Vienna Woods or the surrounding country. Only on one Sunday during the three and a half months for which the diary entries are available is he unable to get to the 'Eisernes Tor' although the weather is beautiful. On Wednesday, 9 February Julie and the servants are at the Opera-Redoute (a masked ball held during Carnival time), but less than two weeks later an entry reads 'Julie has attempted suicide'. (Dr August Ungethüm thought that the cause was disappointment in love.) Several entries later refer to her serious illness which is diagnosed as galloping phthisis. She must have made a good recovery because she died only a few years ago.

In his earlier years Wagner-Jauregg was very keen on athletics, performing regular callisthenics and weight-lifting. He was also keen on riding – M. Gerstmann mentioned that her husband often joined him and Julie on their rides in the Prater. However, his great love was walking and mountaineering which he only abandoned when in his late years his health became precarious. Among his leisure activities were Tarok, a popular card game in Austria, and chess. M. Gerstmann records her visit to the Circus in company with her husband and Wagner-Jauregg. He evidently loved the Circus.

There is no evidence that Wagner-Jauregg took much interest in the very lively artistic life that flourished in Vienna at the turn of the century. His name does not occur in accounts of developments in the arts, literature and music in which the names of other medical men figure. Among the surviving letters there is one from Wagner-Jauregg to the well-known pianist Alfred Grünfeld (1852–1924), (the original of the letter is in the Library of the City and Province of Vienna – Wiener Stadt- und Landesbibliothek) asking him to perform at an evening function in support of Mensa Academica in March 1908, which was clearly occasioned by a charitable cause. Also there is a letter from a university choral society saying how pleased they were that Wagner-Jauregg had decided to rejoin the society in which he had spent his youth. He must, therefore, have been musical, although he never mentions music in his *Memoirs*. There was a piano in his apartment and Hermann v. Schmeidel, a second cousin (he calls himself his nephew, as is the custom in Austria) who, as a music student, lived with Wagner-Jauregg for five years, tells how early every morning he would be woken up by a chord struck on the piano by his 'uncle' and asked what chord it was. Fortunately, Hermann had absolute pitch and had no difficulty in answering the question. Evidently, Wagner-Jauregg's maxim was 'He who sleeps, works and experiences little'.

During the last years of his life Wagner-Jauregg suffered from ill-health. In the letter to the University of Edinburgh in which he apologised for not being able to travel to Scotland to receive the Cameron Prize, he said that for the past eight years he had been suffering from atrial fibrillation and recently had had repeated attacks of lung infarction which caused high temperatures and forced him to stay in bed. In a letter to Paul de Kruif, dated August 1935, he said that he was gliding down the life line, at times quickly, at others more slowly and that he had now reached the zone where Men Against Death could no longer do anything.

However, in the draft of a letter to Adolf Lorenz, dated 30 January 1939, he said that, for the time being, he was not able to heed Lorenz's warning to free himself from chasing spirochaetes as he wanted to die in the saddle. Speaking of his faith, he wrote 'I have long been convinced that man is the most conceited of all living creatures that cannot resign himself to the thought of the destruction of the individual through death and deludes himself with words like immortality and beyond. I do not believe that dogs and horses, animals that are most alike men mentally, have these worries. Therefore I do not say meet you again in the beyond but faithful friendship until the end.'

H. Hoff writes in an article on Wagner-Jauregg 'I know little about the death of Wagner-Jauregg. Probably he, who gave health to so many and had understanding for so many, died a lonely man.' It is true that, when he died on 27 September 1940, he was living on his own. Many of his former assistants and colleagues must have emigrated and his son lived in Frankfurt, but his step-daughter and his wife were in Vienna and the author has been told that they visited him often. The last entry in his Diary – which is very empty compared with the entries for part of 1920 – refers to someone who was coming to repair the stove.

Honours and tributes

Towards the end of his life Wagner-Jauregg was showered with honours, some of which have already been mentioned. In 1907 he was awarded the title of 'Hofrat' (Councillor), a title similar to a knighthood in England, usually conferred on heads of large institutions. Besides receiving the Nobel Prize, the Erb-medal, the Cameron Prize for 1935, Honorary Doctorates of Philosophy and of Law, he was made an Honorary Member of the Austrian Academy of Science in 1929 and Honorary Citizen of Vienna and of Wels (his birthplace). When he retired in 1928 one of the Vienna medical weeklies, the *Wiener Medizinische Wochenschrift*, published a whole issue as a Festschrift in his honour and in 1937 on the occasion of his 80th birthday the other weekly, the *Wiener Klinische Wochenschrift*, dedicated a number to him as a birthday gift. A large photograph adorns the first page and the number is introduced by a distinguished colleague, the Editor of the periodical and his successor at the Clinic, O. Pötzl. In a later issue there is a detailed survey of his work by the Hungarian professor, L. Benedek, Director of the Neurology Clinic at Budapest. On his 80th birthday Wagner-Jauregg became Honorary President of the Vienna Medical Society and also of the Society for Psychiatry and Neurology of Vienna, which also struck a medal and founded a lecture named after him. He was awarded Honorary Doctorates in Philosophy and Law of the University of Vienna and he received the Honorary Badge for Art and Science.

After his death a bust was placed in the forecourt of the University of Vienna and a plaque attached to the building in which he lived for most of his adult life. The City of Vienna named a large municipal building project after him. On the anniversary of his 100th birthday, in 1957, the Austrian National Bank printed his portrait on the 500 schilling bank note. It also appeared in the same year on the 2.40 schilling stamp. As recently as 1970 the neurological hospital in Linz, the second largest city in Austria, was renamed the Oberösterreichische Landes-Nervenklink Wagner-Jauregg, another proof that at least in Austria Wagner-Jauregg's name is still remembered.

SUMMING UP

To appreciate Wagner-Jauregg's significance in the history of medicine, it must be remembered that until nearly the end of the nineteenth century fascination with diagnosis and neglect of therapy characterized the Vienna Medical Faculty. According to William Johnston, by 1850, scepticism toward traditional therapy had so taken root that the only medicament used in the General Hospital was cherry brandy. This attitude reached a peak of intensity under Carl von Rokitansky and Joseph Skoda, who both insisted that diagnosis came first. Only mechanical and external intervention were considered as efficacious, internal therapy being a superstition with no scientific basis. A. Kussmaul, a German physician who came to Vienna in 1847 to attend a post-graduate course, wrote very scathingly about this attitude. According to him, teachers and pupils forgot that the task of medicine is healing. Things had reached the point where some young doctors awaited with greater interest the outcome of an autopsy than the success of their therapy.

However, even before the end of the century, some medical men had begun to counteract this therapeutic nihilism, and Wagner-Jauregg was one of the first to develop therapies that actually cured many who had been thought to be hopeless cases. His malaria therapy brought thousands back to health and his realisation of the importance of thyroid hormone in the prevention and treatment of cretinism restored many children to a normal life. His campaign for goitre prophylaxis, although only temporarily successful, paved the way for the prevention of a wide-spread illness in the alpine districts.

Although Wagner-Jauregg's name has been largely forgotten now and gets little mention in psychiatric textbooks, it ought to be remembered that at the time his work brought health to thousands and alleviated the sufferings of many. It was not knowledge for its own sake that he sought, but knowledge that might benefit humanity. Throughout his scientific work, his constant endeavour was to find a successful therapy.

BIBLIOGRAPHY

This final chapter is largely based on archival material at the Institut für Geschichte der Medizin der Universität Wien, the first chapter of Theodor Wagner-Jauregg's autobiography *Mein Lebensweg als bioorganischer Chemiker* (Stuttgart: Wissenschaftliche Verlagsgesellschaft, 1985) and his article in *Die Presse*, 3.3.1957, pp. 17–18, interviews with Professor Theodor Wagner-Jauregg (d. 1992) and Julius Wagner-Jauregg's stepgrandsons, Dr August Ungethüm (d. 1990) and Dipl. Ing. Ernst Ungethüm (d. 1992). Other sources consulted are listed below.

Gerstmann, M. *Proc.Virchow-Pirquet Medical Society*, 1979, 33: 48–49.

Hoff, Hans. *Wien.Klin.Wschr.*, 1950, 62: 888–889.

Jenner, F.A. 'Erwin Stengel. A personal memoir.' In: *150 Years of British Psychiatry*. Ed. Berrios and Freeman. London: Royal College of Psychiatry, 1992, p. 437.

Johnston, William M. *The Austrian Mind*. Berkeley: University of California Press, 1972.

Kussmaul, A. *Jugenderinnerungen eines alten Arztes*. Stuttgart: 1899.

Memorial Meeting. *Wien.Med.Wschr.*, 1940, 90: no. 44, 844.

Schmeidel, Hermann von. *Tagespost* (Graz), 11.3.1937.

Schnitzler, Artur. *Jugend in Wien*. Wien: 1968.

Stransky, E. *Selbstbiographie*. MS held at the Institut für Geschichte der Medizin der Universität Wien: *Wien.Klin.Wschr.*, 1957, 69: 177–178.

Thury, Elizabeth. *Weltpresse*, no. 100, 1951.

Wagner-Jauregg, Julius. *Lebenserinnerungen.* Ed. L. Schönbauer and M. Jantsch. Wien: Springer Verlag, 1950.

Wagner-Jauregg's Eightieth Birthday Celebrations. *Wien.Klin.Wschr.,* 1937, 50: 275–362.

Wagner-Jauregg's Retirement. *Wien.Med.Wschr.,* 1928, 78: 891 et seq.

Wagner-Jauregg Lecture and Medal. *Die Presse,* 10.3.1987, article originally published in *Neue Freie Presse,* March 1937.

Appendix

In the Footsteps of Wagner-Jauregg: the Horton Malaria Laboratory
by Henry R. Rollin MD, FRCP, FRCPsych (Hon), FRCPsych, DPM

On the 1 January 1913, of 103 842 patients suffering from mental disorder in 95 public mental hospitals in England, 6380 (5352 men and 1028 women) were diagnosed as suffering from general paralysis of the insane (GPI). In the mental hospitals administered by the London County Council at that time more than eight per cent of new admissions were found to be suffering from the same dread disease, a syphilitic invasion of the brain and central nervous system, most of whom were doomed to die a wretched, lingering death. There was no known cure. There was no hope.

These few statistics serve to throw into relief the hugely important work carried out in the Horton Malaria Laboratory and, coincidentally, the incalculable contribution of Wagner-Jauregg towards the amelioration of human suffering. Indeed, the story to be unfolded may read like science fiction, but it is nonetheless a fascinating chapter of science fact.

The prologue is staged in Austria where in 1917 Julius Wagner-Jauregg, Professor of Psychiatry and Neurology at the University of Vienna, was able to induce malaria in GPI victims with dramatically successful effects on the course of their existing disease.

News of this epoch-making advance in treatment spread rapidly throughout the civilised world, but the First World War of 1914 – 18 and its aftermath delayed its introduction in the UK. It was not in fact until 1922 that the first patients were inoculated with malaria in England. The pioneer in this instance was Professor Warrington Yorke (1883 – 1943) who had access to patients at the Whittingham Mental Hospital located near Liverpool.

An account of this historic event is contained in the Ninth Report of the Board of Control 1923 (for the year 1922), p. 81. It reads:

The Treatment of General Paralysis of the Insane

(a) By inoculation of Malaria Parasites (Wagner-Jauregg method of treatment). Following the reports of various Continental writers of the very favourable results obtained by inoculation of general paralysis of the insane with malaria parasites, it was decided to try this form of treatment in a number of cases of general paresis in this Institution.

On July 21st, 1922, three male cases of general paralysis were inoculated subcutaneously with blood obtained by venous puncture from a patient suffering from malaria fever. After an incubation period of 16 days in one instance, and of 21 days in another, malaria parasites were detected in the blood of two of the cases, and attacks of malaria fever appeared.

It is worthy of mention that in the same year some of the earliest attempts at malaria therapy in neuro-syphilis were carried out by Colonel S.P. James FRS (1870 – 1946) at the Manor War Hospital, Epsom, adjoining Horton Hospital. In 1923 more hospitals, including some of the London County mental hospitals, adopted the Wagner-Jauregg treatment. In 1925, however, an important landmark was reached: by arrangement with the Ministry of Health, the Board of Control and the London County Council, a centre exclusively for the application of malaria therapy to cases of general paralysis, with a laboratory for the specialist study of malaria *per se*, was established at Horton Hospital, Epsom, the first of its sort to be set up in the UK and possibly in the world. It was first known as 'C' Hospital, but the name changed to the Horton Malaria Laboratory, then to the Mott Clinic (in memory of Sir Frederick Mott (1853 – 1926), director of the Central Laboratory and Pathologist to the L.C.C. mental hospitals) and Malaria Reference Laboratory and the W.H.O. Regional Malaria Centre for Europe.

Irrespective of the name-tag attached to it, the clinic flourished. An index of its value is seen in the fact that at Horton Hospital alone some 10 000 patients underwent treatment by induced malaria apart, that is, from the provision of infective material from the laboratory for inoculating cases in different centres throughout the British Isles and Europe.

The recovery rate stood at from 30 to 40 per cent, but it soon became apparent that the degree of recovery depended on how early the treatment was given, that is, how soon before irreversible damage had been done to the brain. For the rest, the best that could be hoped for was the arrest of the destructive process. But hope in varying degrees could be offered where previously there was none.

Under its director, Colonel S.P. James, who had crossed the boundary fence between the Manor and Horton hospitals, a steady stream of publications began to appear in scientific journals all over the world bearing the imprint of the Horton Laboratory. In particular help of inestimable value to the Allied cause was contributed by the laboratory in the Second World War.

Top priority was given to the further development of the drug, mepacrine, already known to be more effective than quinine as a curative agent. It fell to the Horton Laboratory to test the drug which because of its potential importance, necessitated conditions of maximum security. The ultimate success of this particular research programme is in itself a story of epic proportions.

Indeed the history of the Horton Laboratory is remarkable involving as it does the work of J.A. Sinton VC, FRS, Major General Sir Gordon Covell and P.C.C. Garnham FRS, and above all that of P.G. Shute—who like Colonel James had previously worked at the Manor Hospital—ably assisted by Miss Marjorie Maryon. There he had joined Sir Ronald Ross, the Nobel Laureate, after war service in which he had contributed enormously to the treatment of malaria on the battlefield. The story of the Horton Laboratory and later Horton Malaria Reference Laboratory has been briefly and inadequately told elsewhere (Rollin, Henry R: Epsom Med Soc Trans 1981 – 86, pp. 18 – 19).

INDEX

W-J stands for Julius Wagner-Jauregg

Abraham, Karl (1877 – 1925) 106
aconite for trigeminal neuralgia, W-J's
    treatment 182
Adamkiewicz, Albert (1850 – 1921) 35
addicts, W-J's tactics 65
Adler, Alfred (1870 – 1937) 112
Adler, Friedrich (b. 1879) 89 – 90
Adler, Victor (1852 – 1918) 89, 90
ageing and longevity 192 – 3
agoraphobia, W-J's treatment 65
Albrecht, O. 3
alcohol
    misuse 62
    toxicology 96
alcoholics, institutions for,
    W-J's report to Senior Health Council
        39, 65
    W-J's tactics 65
alcoholism in relation to the insane 96
Alexander, F. 113
Alexander, Gustav (1873 – 1932) 127
alpine goitre, see goitre
amentia 64
American Journal of Psychiatry on malaria
    therapy 166
amnesia, retroactive, after resuscitation,
    W-J's research 47
Amrush, Emil (d. 1919) 29
anaesthesia, by cocaine 35, 108
animal experiments 27
    excision of thyroid gland 35, 117 – 19
    function of glands in relation to
        circulatory system 108
    on cutting through nerves in pyramidal
        tract 59 – 60
    to test effect of thyroid medication 131
    W-J's 15, 27 – 8, 35, 59, 117 – 19
anopheles mosquitoes
    on banks of Danube 162
    search for at asylum 160
    transmission of induced malaria 165,
        170

anthrax, effect on GPI 152
antibiotics viii, 1
antiluetic medication, *see* iodine; mercury;
        neosalvarsan;
    salvarsan
Anton, Gabriel (1858 – 1933) 66 – 7
Arlt, Ferdinand von (1812 – 87) 19
Army hospital, neurology department,
    W-J assists 101
Arzt, Leopold (b. 1883) 199
Asylum of Lower Austria (*see also*
        Psychiatric Clinic, First) 33 – 4, 55
    move to Steinhof 61, 68
asylums
    admission to 91, 93, 95, 97
    voluntary entry to 97
ataxia 188
Austria, break up of Empire 104
Austrian Office of Public Health 138, 139
Austrian Society for Health Care, goitre
        prevention 131, 138
Autenrieth's ointment 154

bacillus pyocyaneus to produce fever
        156 – 7
bacterial proteins in fever therapy 156 – 7
bacteriology, Stricker's attitude 29
Bamberger, Heinrich (1822 – 88) 13, 15,
        19, 30, 110
    lectures and clinics 13, 18, 26, 31, 60
    W-J at Bamberger's Clinic 30 – 31, 36
bank note forger, W-J's evidence 88 – 9
Barzillai-Vivaldi, G. 165
Basedow
    affected by heredity 189
    caused by iodine 139, 140
Bauer, Otto (1882 – 1938) 111
Baumann, E. (1846 – 96) 131
Bayard, O. (1812 – 52) 139, 145
Beer, H.H. (1798 – 1873) 91
Belgium, King of (Leopold II) 24
Benedek, L. 203
Benedikt, Moriz (1835 – 1920) 88, 93, 95
Bering, Professor 173

Bernheim, H. (1840 – 1919) 182
Billroth, Theodor von (1829 – 94) 13, 15,
    18, 21, 118
biology, subject in examination 77
Bircher, E. (b. 1882) 132, 140, 141,
    143 – 7
Bircher, H. (1850 – 1923) 123, 124
bismogenol 171
bladder, innervation, W-J's paper 49
blood groups, importance in malaria
    therapy 170
blood pressure measurements
    W-J's experiments 26 – 7, 28
blood transfusions to cure psychoses 153
Boeck, Ernst (1857 – 1924) 59, 60,
    156 – 7
Boerhaave, Hermann (1668 – 1745) 9,
    151
Bosnia and Herzegovina, Austrian
    involvement 17
Bourneville, D.M. (1840 – 1909) 124
Boussingault, J.B. (1801 – 87) 138
brain, W-J's investigations
    anatomy 34
    blood circulation 37
Breitner, Burghard (b. 1884) 2
Bright, Richard (1789 – 1858) 30
Bright's disease 30
Brown-Sequard, C.E. (1817 – 94) 181
Brücke, Ernst von (1819 – 92) 12, 29,
    108, 109
Brugsch, Theodor (1878 – 1963) 156
Bühler, Karl (1879 – 1963) 183
Bulgaria, King of (Ferdinand) 35 – 6
Burroughs Wellcome, suppliers of thyroid
    tablets 126, 127, 129

Cachexia strumipriva 117
Cameron Prize 172, 202
carbohydrate metabolism and melancholia
    64
cataract, combination with muscular
    dystrophy 189
Charcot, Jean-Martin (1825 – 93) 36, 47,
    108, 109, 110
Chatin, G.A. (1813 – 1901) 137
cholera, effect on psychoses 151, 153
cocaine anaesthesia
    in eye operations: priority dispute 108
    W-J's research 35
Cohnheim, Julius (1839 – 84) 29
Coindet, J.F. (1774 – 1834) 137
Commission to investigate treatment of
    war neuroses 105 – 7
    Freud's evidence 106 – 7

Report 107
congenital diseases, W-J on 188-9
Congress on Tuberculosis 156
Conrad, Eugen 35
controlled trials 167
Covell, Sir Gordon 209
cretinism (*see also* deaf-mutism; iodine;
        thyroid gland;
        thyroidal theory; thyroid therapy)
    difficulty in diagnosis 121 – 2
    imbecility 132
    in Hungary and Galicia 125
    in Styria 119 – 21
    Institution to study 130
    need for early diagnosis 131
    sporadic and endemic, comparison of
        symptoms 132
    W-J's statistical studies 120 – 21
    W-J's study xiv, xv, 1, 49, 117 – 35
criminality arising from pathological
        causes 98, 186
criminally insane, institutions for, W-J's
        plea 93 – 4, 95 – 6, 99
curare used in animal experiments 27
Czermak, Johann (1828 – 73) 43

Danzig goitre 142
Dattner, Bernhard 164
de Kruif, Paul 3, 171 – 2, 201
deaf-mutism of cretins 121, 122-3, 127,
    132
degenerates and paralytics, comparison
    186
degeneration ix, 62, 185
degree ceremony, University of Vienna
    23
delirium alcoholicum 96
dementia paralytica, *see* GPI
dementia praecox *see* schizophrenia
dentistry in medical curriculum 77
depression, a body problem 63 – 4
dermatology in medical curriculum
    45 – 6, 77
Deutsch, Helene (1884 – 1982) 3, 49, 63,
    64, 101 – 2, 111
diabetes insipidus 37
diabetes mellitus, affected by heredity 189
diagnostics, development by Vienna
    School 9 – 10
diathermal treatment as alternative to
    malaria therapy 171, 172
diminished responsibility, W-J's proposal
    98
Diviak, R. 126, 131, 137
Doerr, R. (1871 – 1952) 162

Donath, Julius (1870 – 1950) 79
Durig, Arnold (b. 1872) 183
Duchek, A. (1824 – 82) 19, 31
Dumreicher, Johann von (1815 – 80) 13,
    14
dysthymia neuralgica transitoria 37

Economo, Constantin von (1876 – 1931)
    xvii, 198
Eggenberger, Hans (1881 – 1946) 141
Egypt, occupied by British 25
Ehrenhaft, Felix (1879 – 1952) 183
Eissler, K.R. Comments on Commission
    proceedings 105 – 7
  on Freud 110, 111
electric torture accusation 105
electrotherapy 103 – 7
Ellenberger, Henri F. 2
Elzholz, Adolf (1863 – 1925) 60, 88
Emperor's ring, W-J's failure to qualify
    20
encephalitis lethargica, diseases following,
    fever therapy 179, 180
endemic goitre, *see* goitre
Engelskjön's electrodiagnostic examination:
  W-J's criticism 35
epilepsy
    among degenerates 187
    caused by head injury 37
    effect of heredity 189
    effect of intermittent fever 252;
      malaria 151, 152
    Redlich specialist in treatment 60
    role of environmental factors 190
Erb medal 168, 202
erysipelas, effect on insanity 38, 151, 152,
    153
Escherich, Theodor (1857 – 1911) 45, 49,
    155, 196
eugenics, W-J's reflections on xv, 5,
    190 – 2
Eugenics Society, Austrian, W-J
    President 191
Ewald, C.A. (1845 – 1915) 123
examinations
    organisation, Vienna University 74
    regulations, Graz University 45;
      Vienna University 10 – 11
exanthemata, acute, effect on psychoses
    151, 152, 153
extrapyramidal tract, discovery 59

Fahrmann, Dr. 101
Faradism, *see* electrotherapy
Feldhof Asylum 43, 44

outings to 45
Fellenberg, T. von 141, 144
Ferstel, Marie, Baroness 111
fever, effect on polyneuritis 63; on
    psychoses (W-J's study)
    38, 59, 151 – 5
fever therapy (*see also* bacterial proteins;
    malaria therapy;
    rat bite fever; recurrent fever;
    tuberculin; vaccine treatment)
  nervous diseases 179, 180
  Rosenblum's experiments 154 – 5
  W-J's work 151 – 5, 179 – 80; collected
    papers 173
Fick, Adolf (1829 – 1901) 28
First Word War, effect on Clinic 101 – 3
Flück, W. 141
Forel, August (1848 – 1931) 96, 187
forensic evidence: Krafft-Ebing's 83 – 5;
    Wagner-Jauregg's 83 – 90
  case of bank note forger 88 – 9
  case of medical student thief 84
  Girardi affair 85 – 8
  Prime Minister's murder 89 – 90
forensic psychiatry, W-J's work 83 – 100
formes frustes 188
Francis Joseph, Emperor (1830 – 1916) 87
Francois II 181
Freud, Sigmund (1856 – 1939) (*see also*
    psychoanalysis)
  as expert witness 106
  astonished at results of W-J's animal
    experiments 60
  at Stricker's Institute 108
  awarded Venia legendi in neurology
    108
  awarded titles of professor 110 – 11
  criticized by Raimann 112
  exchange of letters with W-J 113 – 14
  loses facilities at Meynert's Clinic 109
  praises Charcot on hysteria 109 – 10
  refuses to rule out hypnotism 109
  sets up in practice 109
  studies under Charcot 108, 109
  transferred from Neurology
    Department 109
  W-J, relations with, xv, 108 – 9,
    112 – 13
  W-J reports on 111
Freud's theory, *see* psychoanalysis
Freud, Frau Dr. 101
Freund, Leopold (1868 – 1943) 79
Friedländer, Friedrich 158
Friedreich, Nikolaus (1826 – 82) 254
Friedreich's ataxia 188

Frohnleiten, district of Styria, cretinism
119, 120
fuchsin tests by W-J 30
Fuchs, Alfred (1870 – 1927) 102, 160
Fuchs, Ernst (1851 – 1930) 36, 75

GPI (general paralysis of the insane)
diagnosis 157, 158
effect of anthrax 152; malaria, *see*
malaria therapy; smallpox 152;
staphylococci 159; suppuration
152 – 4; tuberculin q.v.
in London hospitals
mercury, iodine and salvarsan in
treatment 158, 160, 164, 167
need for early treatment 170 – 71, 209
Spirochaetes in brain of paralytics 168,
171
treatment by X-rays 173
Gadelius, Bror (1862 – 1938) 169
Galen 151, 181
Garnham, P.C.C. 209
Gärtner, Gustav (1855 – 1937) 14, 37, 50
gastrointestinal troubles, relation with
psychoses 63
Gauster, Moriz (1828 – 96) 57, 58, 61
general paralysis of the insane, *see* GPI
genetics (*see also* heredity): W-J's
reflections) xv, 5
Gerhardt, Karl (1833 – 1902) 31
German Society for Internal Medicine
(Deutscher Verein für Innere
Medizin), AGM April 1906, 129;
Wiesbaden 1926, 167
German Society for Psychiatry (Deutscher
Verein für
Psychiatrie) 163, 165, 169
Gerstmann, Josef (b. 1887) 163
Gerstmann, M. 199, 201
Gestapo 200
Gicklhorn, J. and R. 110 – 11
Girardi, Alexander (1850 – 1918) 85 – 8,
91
glands, function, in relation to circulatory
system 108
goitre (*see also* goitre prophylaxis)
aetiology 139, 145 – 6
endemic: symptom of cretinism 122,
123 – 4, 137
Danzig goitre 142
iodine deficiency as cause 145
iodine treatment 142 – 3
relation with cretinism 131
sporadic 123 – 4
goitre prophylaxis (*see also* salt: iodization)

results 142 – 3
role of iodine 1, 131, 138
W-J's achievements xiv, xv, 1
W-J's campaign 137 – 49
W-J's reviews of progress 146
Gomperz, Elise 111
Gonda, V.E. 155
Graz, Asylum and Psychiatric Clinic 44,
45, 155
Graz, general hospital, W-J chief medical
officer 45
Graz, University 43
Graz, W-J in 43 – 53
Griesinger, Wilhelm (1817 – 68) 37, 39
Grünfeld, Alfred (1852 – 1924) 201

Hainisch, Marianne (1839 – 1936) 191
Halban, H. von (1870 – 1926) 66
Hamburg Asylum introduces malaria
therapy 165
Handbook of Psychiatry, ed. Aschaffenburg
W-J critical 158; W-J on thyroidal
theory 132
Hartmann, Friedrich (b. 1871) 81
head injury: cause of epilepsy 37;
insanity 37
heart, accelerating nerves, W-J's paper 15
hebephrenia, treatment 181
Hebra, Ferdinand von (1816 – 80) 10
heredity
effect on Basedow 189; on diabetes
189;
on mental illness 162, 185, 189; on
nervous diseases 189
statistical methods 187
Hippocrates 151, 181
histology, separate subject 77
Hitler, Adolf (1889 – 1945) 199
Hitzig, Eduard (1838 – 1907) 50
Hochenegg, Julius von (1859 – 1940) 68
Hochstetter, F. von (1861 – 1954) 63
Hoff, H. (1897 – 1969) xiv, xvi, 99, 202
Hoffmann, Dr. 85 – 8
Hoffmann, Erich (1868 – 1959) 173
Hofmann, Eduard von (1827 – 97) 39,
76, 92
Högler, F. 144
Holl, Moriz (1852 – 1920) 40, 49, 117
Holub, Emil (1847 – 1902) 24
Holzknecht, Guido (1872 – 1931) 79
Homer 181
hormonal therapy 180 – 81
Horton Hospital, Epsom, uses malaria
therapy 166, 208
Horton Malaria Laboratory 208

Huntington, George Sumner
(1850 – 1916) 188
Huntington's chorea 188
Hunziker, Hans (1878 – 1941) 141
hydrorhoea nasalis 181
hyperthyroidism caused by iodine 139,
140, 142, 144 – 5, 189
hypnotism 182
use by Freud 109
Hyrtl, Joseph (1810 – 94) 10
hysteria: diagnosis by W-J 36
hysteria, male, Freud's paper 109 – 10

I.G. Farben, maker of stovarsol 172
imbecility, due to malfunction of thyroid
132
impotence, treatment 181
infectious diseases, effect on insanity, W-
J's study 38, 59,
151 – 5; relation with polyneuritis 63
Innsbruck university, W-J recommended
for post 40
insane
care and protection 91, 93, 95
criminals 94 – 5
guardianship 93
insanity (*see also* psychiatric disorders)
caused by alcoholism 62, 96; head
injury 37; neuralgia 37
cured after attempted suicide 47
effect of fever 38, 59, 151 – 5
legislation xiv, xv, 1, 90 – 99
insanity defence 98
Institute for Children's Diseases 109
Institute for Physiology 108
Institute for General and Experimental
Pathology (Stricker's
Institute) 29
appointment of Director 80
foundation 9
Freud and W-J at 108
W-J at 14 – 15, 18, 19, 23, 25 – 9, 31,
108
Institute of Pathological Anatomy, *see*
Institute for General and
Experimental Pathology
Institute of Radiology, proposal 80
interdiction 90, 93, 97
law 99
intermittent fevers
effect on epilepsy 152
effect on psychoses 151, 153
internal medicine, thought processes
introduced into psychiatry by W-J
xiv, xv, 48, 63

internal medicine, Clinics for, *see*
Bamberger; Nothnagel
International Goitre Conference, 1927:
141; 1938: 147
International Medical Congress, Budapest
1909 158
International Neurological Congress, 1935
155
iodine (*see also* hyperthyroidism; salt:
iodization)
content passed in urine 141
in GPI treatment 142 – 3
necessary for thyroid function 1,
131 – 2, 137 – 8, 145
treatment 142 – 3

Jaksch, Rudolf von (1855 – 1947) 31
James, S.P. (1870 – 1946) 208, 209
Jewish students, proposed reduction of
number 77 – 8
Jews, W-J's attitude to xv – xvi,
198 – 200
John, Dr. 198
Joseph II (1741 – 90) 9, 55
Judenburg (Carinthia), W-J's activities
126

Karplus, I.P. (1866 – 1936) 3, 62
Kaspar, F. 141
Kasparek, Dr. 58 – 9
Kauders, Joseph Vincenz (1850 – 1916)
30
Kauders, O. (1893 – 1949) 165, 167
Kauders, Walter 105
kidney, removal, effect 118 – 19
Kienböck, Robert (1871 – 1953) 79
Kiernan, J.G. (1800 – 74) 153
Kimball, O.P. 137
Klinger, R. 138
Knoll's polygraph 31
Koch, Robert (1843 – 1910) 29, 156
Kocher, Theodor (1841 – 1917) 117, 122,
123
Königstein, Leopold (1850 – 1924) 108
Köstl, Franz (1811 – 82) 43, 138, 153
Koller, Jenny 187
Koller, Karl (1851 – 1946) 35, 108
Kornfeld, Adolf (1861 – 1938) 69, 81
Kozlowski, M. 107
Kraepelin, Emil (1856 – 1926) 64, 69, 189
Krafft-Ebing, Richard von (1840 – 1902)
xv, 39 – 40, 44, 50, 51, 62,
92, 111, 187
Director of Graz Asylum 44
Director of First Psychiatric Clinic 39;

at Second Clinic 50, 57
forensic activities 83 – 5
health 66, 84
on insanity legislation 92 – 3
on Vienna Clinics 58, 67
Kraus, F. (1858 – 1936) 127, 129
Kremer, Alfred, Freiherr von (1828 – 89)
   16, 25
Kretschmer, Ernst (1888 – 1964) xvi, 190
Kundrat, Hans (1845 – 93) 38, 76
Kussmaul, Adolf (1822 – 1902) 10, 14,
   203
Kusy, Emanuel, Ritter von Dubrav
   (1844 – 1905) 125, 127
Kutschera, Dr. 129, 130
Kyrle, Josef (1880 – 1926) 164 – 5

Lakarski, Josef (1854 – 1924) 25 – 6, 28
Land, Victor von (1838 – 1921) 10
Lang, Donat (d. 1872) 43
laryngology in medical syllabus 77
Last, S.L. (1902 – 91) 2, 63, 65, 102
Lehrbuch der Organotherapie, W-J's chapter on
   thyroid 132
Leidesdorf, Max (1818 – 89) xv, 32, 36,
   48, 51, 55 – 7, 62
   blood transfusion experiment 153
   heart attack 38 – 9, 153
   funeral 40
   suggests thyroid excision 35, 117 – 18
   supports W-J 109
Lesky, E. 56
Leyden, Ernst von (1832 – 1910) 31
Lipp, Eduard (1831 – 91) 45
Lister, Joseph (1786 – 1869) 13, 14
Lloyds Office, W-J wants to apply for
   cruise 23 – 4
Life span, human 192 – 3
Lombroso, Cesare (1835 – 1909) xv, 62,
   185, 186
Lorenz, Adolf (1854 – 1946) 10, 198, 202
Ludwig, Karl (1816 – 95) 15
Lueger, Karl (1844 – 1910) 61, 198
lumbar puncture, *see* Wassermann test
lunacy laws, *see* insanity: legislation

malaria (*see also* intermittent fevers; malaria
   therapy; quinine)
   effect on epilepsy 151, 152; on
     psychoses 155
   induced v. true 166
   tertiana 161, 162, 163; change into
     quotidian 170
   transmission by anopheles mosquitoes
     165, 170

tropica 162, 163
malaria therapy
   blood groups important in therapy 170
   compared to recurrent fever therapy
     167 – 8
   danger of infecting medical staff 165,
     170
   effect: due to fever or increased
     resistance 171
   in England 207 – 9
   method of infection 166
   W-J's work xiii, xiv, xv, 1, 159 – 65,
     170 – 3
   world-wide 165 – 9
manic-depressive psychoses (*see also*
   melancholia) 63 – 4
   effect of heredity 189
   fever therapy 179
Manor War Hospital 208
Maresch, Rudolf (1868 – 1936) 81
Maria Theresa, Empress (1717 – 1780) 9,
   90
Marie, Pierre (1853 – 1940) 188
Marie's ataxia 188
Marine, David (1880 – 1976) 137
Martini, Erich (b. 1880) 170
marriage between relatives 190
marriage counselling 190
Maryon, Marjorie 209
masturbation, treatment 181
Mauthner, Ludwig (1840 – 94) 154
medical education, further, 76, 81
Medical Society of Styria (Verein der
   Aerzte in Steiermark) 45, 46
   Communications 122, 128
Medical Society of Vienna, *see* Vienna
   Medical Society
medical syllabus, revision 45 – 6, 76 – 7
medulla oblongata, W-J's study 37
melancholia
   and carbohydrate metabolism 64
   effect of malaria 151
Men against Death (Paul de Kruif) 3, 201
Menger, Anton (1841 – 1906) 75
Mendel, J.G. (1822 – 84) 187, 188
meningitis, non-tubercular, fever therapy
   179, 180
mental illness, *see* insanity; psychiatric
   disorders
mepacrin 209
mercury in GPI treatment 158, 164
Merke, F. 146
Meyer, Ernst (1871 – 1931) 158
Meyer, Ludwig (1827 – 1900) 154
Meynert, Theodor (1833 – 92) xiv, xvi,

32, 36, 38, 51, 56 – 7, 62, 187
amentia 64
  on W-J's application 36
  on W-J's diagnosis 36
  on W-J's paper 48
  relation with Freud 109, 110
migraine, degenerative, treatment 181
Moebius, P.J. (1853 – 1907) 47 – 8, 186
Morel, Benedict (1809 – 73) xv, 62, 185
Mott, Sir Frederick (1853 – 1926) 208
Mott Clinic 208
Motschukoffsky, J. 153, 155
movement disorders, caused by shell-
  shock 103 – 4
Müller, Johannes (1801 – 58) 12, 29
multiple sclerosis: fever therapy 179, 180
Mundy, J. von (1822 – 94) 91
Murray, G.R. (1865 – 1939) 124, 125
muscular dystrophy
  combined with cataract 189
  effect of heredity 189
  effect of infection 154
mutism (*see also* deaf-mutism) effect of
  shell-shock 103
Myotonoklonia trepidans 103
myxoedema, due to non-function of
  thyroid 123

Naecke, Paul (1851 – 1913) 186
Narrenturm (Fools' Tower) 55
National Socialist Party 199
Nature on malaria therapy 166
neo-salvarsan treatment following malaria
  therapy 161, 162, 164, 171
nervous diseases
  non-syphilitic 179
  somatic origin 63
  W-J's lectures 62
nervus vagus, respiratory activites 15
neuralgia: transitoria 37; trigeminal 182
neurology (*see also* nervous diseases) in
  medical syllabus 77
Neurology Clinic (Second Psychiatric
  Clinic) 57, 102 – 3
neurolues (neuro-syphilis) *see* GPI; tabes
Neusser, Edmund von (1852 – 1912) 35,
  60
New York State Psychiatric Institute
  adopts malaria therapy 166
Neyman, C.A. 154
no-restraint system introduced 55
Nobel Prize for malaria therapy xiv, 1,
  169
non-syphilitic diseases, fever therapy

179 – 180
Nothnagel, Hermann (1841 – 1905) 31,
  79
  Clinic 31, 108
  supports Freud 109, 111

Obersteiner, H. (1847 – 1922) 38, 60
Obersteiner-Redlich theory of the origin of
  tabes 60
occupational therapy, W-J's attitude 65
Oks, B. 153, 154
On the human life span (W-J's last writing)
  192 – 3
Openchowski, Theodor von (1854 – 1914)
  26 – 7
optic nerve atrophy 145; in tabes 168
osteomalacia, relation with mental
  derangement 37 – 8
otology in medical curriculum 77

paediatrics in medical curriculum 45 – 6,
  77
Papal Encyclical, Dec. 1930 191 – 2
paralytics: comparison with degenerates
  186
parathyroid glands
  discovery 119
  effect of removal 119
Parke-Davis, suppliers of thyroid tablets
  127
Parkinsonism 180
Paschkis, Heinrich (1849 – 1923) 35
Pathology, Institute of, *see* Institute for
  General and Experimental Pathology
penicillin, replaced malaria therapy xiv, 1
Pick, Arnold (1851 – 1924) 50
Pilcz, A. (1871 – 1954) 56, 58, 61, 67,
  157, 158, 186
pituitary gland, thyroid therapy 180
Popper, *Sir* Karl (b. 1902) 1
Pötzl, Otto (1877 – 1962) 63, 64, 81, 101,
  102
Prime Minister's murder, W-J's evidence
  89 – 90
prussic acid, effect on animals 26
Psychiatric Clinic, First (Vienna) 44, 50,
  58
  conditions 34
  history 55 – 8
  W-J assistant 32 – 9
  W-J director 51, 58 – 61
Psychiatric Clinic, Second (Vienna) 50,
  56 – 8, 66 – 9
  effect of First World War 101 – 3
  move to Asylum buildings 69

W-J appointed director 66 – 7
psychiatric disorders (*see also* insanity;
    psychoses)
    effect of alcohol 62, 96; heredity 62,
      85, 187
    non-syphilitic 179
    somatic interpretation xiv, xv, 48, 63
    W-J's articles in Medical Encyclopaedia
      49
    W-J's lectures 62
psychiatrists
    attacked 88, 95, 105
    subject to control 93
psychiatry (*see also* psychiatric disorders)
    descriptive movement xiv, xvi
    in medical curriculum 45 – 6, 50, 56,
      76
    pathological-anatomic school xiv, xvi
    tuition, Graz 44
    W-J's articles, 49; contribution xiv,
      63 – 4, 204
psychical experiments 182 – 3
    W-J's reports 184 – 5
psychoanalysis
    attacked at hearing of Commission
      106 – 7
    attitude to, in Vienna 107
    use in war neuroses 106
    W-J's views xvi, 65, 106, 107, 111 – 12
Psychoanalytical Association 113
psychology, practical 64
    W-J's attitude 107
psychoses (*see also* GPI; manic-depressive
    psychoses; schizophrenia)
    effect of fever, *see* fever therapy
    endogenous and exogenous 64
    relation with gastrointestinal troubles
      63; with osteomalacia 37 – 8
    W-J's lectures 62
psychotherapy, W-J's attitude 64 – 5
puerperal fever, Semmelweiss's discovery
    20
pulmonary circulation, measurement of
    blood pressure 27 – 8

Quervain, F. de (1868 – 1940) 141, 143,
    144
quinine in treatment of intermittent fevers
    153; malaria 160, 161, 162, 167, 170

Raab, W. 33, 144, 145
radiologists, W-J's support 79 – 80
Radiology, Institute of 80
radio-thermal treatment 171, 172
Raimann, E. (1872 – 1949) 61, 64, 67,

    106, 112
Ranzoni, Giuseppe Carlo Antonio
    (1711 – 73) 7
rat-bite fever therapy 167
recurrent fever therapy: effect on
    psychoses 153, 155, 161, 162, 167,
      168
Redlich, Emil (1866 – 1930) 60 – 1, 102
responsibility in criminal proceedings
    98 – 99
resuscitation after suicide 46 – 7
    effect on mental illness 47
Reverdin, J.L. (1842 – 1929) 117
Rieder, Jenny 197
Roazen, Paul 49, 63, 101, 111
Rockefeller Foundation 172
Rokitansky, Carl von (1804 – 78) 9, 10,
    15, 29, 56, 203
Rollin, Henry R. 166, 207
Roretz, von 69
Rosenblum, A.S. (1826 – 1902) 153, 154,
    155
Ross, *Sir* Ronald (1857 – 1932) 209
Rothschild, Alfons 102
Rothschild Foundations 102

salicylic acid poisoning 37
salt: iodization, W-J's campaign 138 – 49
    in Austria 139 – 40, 146 – 7
    opposition to 140 – 41, 143 – 5; in
      Austria 140
    results 142 – 3
Salten, Felix (1869 – 1945) 88
salvarsan (*see also* neosalvarsan) following
    malaria therapy 160, 167
Salzer, F.F. (1827 – 90) 18
Sandström, Ivar (1852 – 89) 119
Schauta, Friedrich (1849 – 1919) 20
Schiff, Moritz (1823 – 1926) 118
Schilder, Paul (1886 – 1940) xvi, 102
schizophrenia 18, 64
    effect of heredity 189
    fever therapy 179
Schlagenhaufer, Friedrich (1866 – 1930)
    44, 131
Schlager, Ludwig (1828 – 85) 38, 51, 56,
    91
Schlick, M. (1882 – 1936) 183
Schmarda, Ludwig K. (1819 – 1908) 11
Schmeidel, Hermann von 201
Schnabel, Isidor (1842 – 1908) 45, 74 – 5
Schneider, Rudi and Willy 183
Schnitzler, Arthur (1862 – 1931) 198
Scholz, Franz 109
Scholz, Wilhelm (b. 1864) 127 – 9, 132

Scholz affair 127 – 9
Schottengymnasium 8
Schratt, Katharina (1853 – 1940) 87
Schroeder, Eduard August 94 – 5, 97
Schüle, Heinrich (1840 – 1916) 32
Schwarz, Gotthald (1880 – 1959) 79
Schweighofer, J. 99
Seguin, E. 182
Semmelweis, Ignaz Philipp (1818 – 65) 20
Semon, F. (1849 – 1921) 124
Senior Health Council
  Commission of Enquiry 92
  W-J acts as referee 91 – 2
  W-J's membership xvi, 2, 66, 92, 97,
    179
  W-J's report on alcoholics 39, 65;
    insanity law 96; psychical
    phenomena 184, 185; treatment of
    cretins 125, 126
septicaemia, vaccine treatment 180
seton 154
sex gland therapy 180 – 81
shell-shock treatment 103 – 7
short-wave high frequency 171, 172
Shute, P.J. 209
Simultan Methode (controlled trial), W-J's
    suggestion 167
Sinton, J.A. 209
skin anaesthesia 35
skin diseases, Hebra's course 10
Skoda, Josef (1805 – 81) 9, 203
smallpox: effect on atrophy of optical
    nerve 154; on GPI 152
sneezing, W-J on 181
snuff tobacco to produce sneezing 181
Society for Psychiatry and Neurology in
    Vienna (Verein für Psychiatrie und
    Neurologie in Wien) 38 – 9, 48, 97,
    181
Society of Asylum Psychiatrists 99
Society of German Neurologists, W-J
    Hon. Member 168
Sölder, Friedrich (1867 – 1943) 102
Späth, J. (1823 – 96) 19 – 20
speech defects
  following shell-shock 103
  improved by malaria therapy 164
Spina, Arnold (1850 – 1918) 29
spinal cord, W-J's research: anatomy 37;
    diseases 35; posterior roots 60;
    pyramidal tract 59 – 60
spinal fluid, analysis (*see also* Wassermann
    test) 168
spirilla, *see* recurrent fever
spirochaetes in brain of paralytics 168,

171
Stanley, H.M. (1841 – 1904) 24
staphylococci: effect on GPI 159;
    meningitis 180; multiple
    sclerosis 180;
Starlinger, J. 59, 60, 99
Staub, H. 113
Steinach, Eugen (1864 – 1944) 181
Stengel, Erwin (1902 – 73) 199
sterilisation 191
stovarsol 172
Stransky, Erwin (1877 – 1962) xiv, xvii,
    1, 106, 199; on psychiatric clinics 58;
    on W-J's appearance and personality
    2, 3, 4, 65, 198; on W-J's lectures
    and views 62, 107, 112
Strasky, Klara 67
streptococci to produce fever 153
Stricker, Salomon (1834 – 98) 14 – 15, 26,
    27, 59
  lectures and teaching methods 15,
    28 – 9
  relations with W-J 28 – 9
  supports W-J 36, 40, 50, 109
  views on bacteriology 29
  W-J at Stricker's Institute 14 – 15, 18,
    19, 23, 25 – 9, 31, 108
Stürgk, Karl, *Graf* (1859 – 1916) 89
Styria: cretinism 119 – 21
Styria, Medical Society of, *see* Medical
    Society of Styria
suppuration: effect on GPI 152; on
    psychoses 154
Svetlin's Institution 86
Swiss Goitre Commission 143
Swiss Medical Weekly (*Schweizerische
    Medizinische Wochenschrift*)
  goitre enquiry 144
Switzerland: use of iodized salt 143
Sydenham, Thomas (1624 – 89) 151
syphilidology in medical curriculum 77
syphilis: elimination 1, 173

tabes
  Obersteiner-Redlich theory 60
  optic atrophy 168
  symptoms and treatment 168
telepathy 182, 183
testicular substances to treat impotence
    181
tetany: result of thyroid excision 118, 119
Thirring, H. 183
Thomson, John (1856 – 1926) 124
Thun, Leo, *Count* (1811 – 88) 8
thyroid gland (*see also* thyroidal theory)

cretinism due to malfunction 1, 118,
122-3
excision 35, 117 – 19
iodine in thyroid function 1, 131 – 2,
137 – 8
thyroid therapy, used by W-J 123,
124 – 30, 180
campaign in Upper Styria 125 – 7
results 129 – 30
tested on dogs 131
thyroidal theory, W-J's 1, 63, 123 – 4,
132; W-J's chapter on 132
Tilkovsky, A. (1871 – 1907) 61, 96
trembling of limbs following shell-shock
103 – 4
trigeminal neuralgia 182
trypanosome gametes 167
tryparsamid 171, 172
tuberculin
effect on psychoses 59, 155 – 9, 164,
167; on schizophrenia 179
toxicity 179
tuberculosis 29, 156
Türkel, Siegfried 92, 94
Türkheim, Ludwig, *Freiherr von*
(1777 – 1846) 9
typhoid: effect on psychoses 151 – 5
typhus: effect on multiple sclerosis 180;
on psychoses 153, 154
typhus vaccine 164, 180

Ungethüm, August (1911 – 90) 197, 200
Ungethüm, Max 197
Ungethüm, Melanie, née Frumkin (d.
1971) 49, 196, 197
urine analysis, fuchsin tests, W-J's 30

vaccination experiments to cure psychoses
153
vaccine treatment 164, 180
van Swieten, Gerard (1700 – 72) 9
vasa deferentia, ligature 181
vasectomies 191
vessiccants 154
Vienna Asylum, *see* Asylum of Lower
Austria
Vienna hospitals: foundation 9
Vienna Medical School 9
Vienna Medical Society (Gesellschaft der
Aerzte in Wien) 9, 82
library 34, 46
W-J at meetings 2, 66, 179
W-J lectures 139, 153 – 4, 182
Vienna Medical Society (after Anschluss
Wiener Medizinische

Gesellschaft)
W-J Memorial Meeting 199
Vienna Psychiatric Clinics, *see* Psychiatric
Clinic First and Second
Vienna University
allocation of candidates for examinations 74 – 5
degree ceremony 23
problems of promotion 78 – 80
professorial board 73 – 82
reduction of student numbers 77 – 8
student unions troubles 75 – 6
W-J Dean of medical faculty 73 – 6
W-J turns down rectorship 80
women: admission to medical study 76
Virchow, Rudolf (1821 – 1902) 9, 13, 156
Vogl, August (1833 – 1909) 25

Wagner, Adolf Johann, later Wagner,
Ritter von Jauregg (1816 – 94) (W-J's
father) 7 – 9, 16, 42
Wagner, Ludovika, née Schmeidel
(1830 – 67) (Adolf's first wife;
W-J's mother) 9
Wagner, Otto (architect) 69
Wagner, Valentin (1785 – 1873) (W-J's
grandfather) 7
Wagner-Jauregg, Anna, née Koch (b.1880)
(W-J's second wife) 196
Wagner-Jauregg, Balbine, née Goldberg,
first married Frumkin
(1862 – 1924) (W-J's first wife) 49,
195 – 6
Wagner-Jauregg, Julie (b. 1900) (W-J's
daughter) 195 – 6, 197, 200
Wagner-Jauregg, Julius (1857 – 1940)
*Life and career**
anecdotes 3 – 4
appearance and dress 2, 3
applies for posts abroad 23, 24 – 5
assistant at First Psychiatric Clinic
32 – 9
at Bamberger's Clinic 30 – 31, 36
at Stricker's Institute 14 – 15, 18, 19,
23, 25 – 9, 31, 108
attends university lectures and clinics
10 – 13, 18, 20
attitude to Jews xv – xvi, 198 – 200
attitude to patients xvi, 3, 5, 65
attitude to students and assistants 4, 60
birth and family background 7
brother 32
Cameron Prize 172, 202
Daughter, pride of 197
Dean of Medical Faculty 73 – 6

death and final illness 201, 202
Director of Graz Psychiatric Clinic 44, 45
Director of First Psychiatric Clinic (Vienna) 51, 58 – 61
Director of Second Psychiatric Clinic (Vienna) 66 – 9
doctor degree awarded 23
emigration plans 23, 24 – 5, 31
Emperor's ring, failure to qualify 20 – 21
Erb medal 168, 202
electric torture accusation 105
exchange of letters with Freud 113 – 14
Eugenics Society, President 191
father, 7, 9, 16, 52; remarries 8
forensic activities 83 – 100
friends 198
German nationalism xv, 198
Graz, Director of Clinic and Chief Medical Officer 43 – 6, 51
health 12, 19, 201
honours and tributes xiv, 1, 168 – 9, 172, 202 – 3
hurt by Freud evidence 106
inaugural lectures 61 – 2, 185, 186 – 7
internal medicine; failure to gain posts ix, 26, 31, 108
lectures 2, 61 – 3, 185, 186 – 7
life style 200 – 202
medical career, choice of 8 – 9
medical syllabus, advocates revision 45 – 6, 76 – 7
military service 15 – 18, 101
mother's death 7, 8, 12
mountaineering and walking activites 12, 49, 200
National Socialism xvii, 199 – 200
Nobel Prize xiv, 1, 169
organisation of further medical education courses 76, 81
personality xvii, 2, 3, 4
private practice xvi, 102
professorships: Graz 43; Vienna 52
psychoanalysis, views on xvi, 106, 111 – 12
relations with Freud xvi, 108 – 9, 112 – 13
relations with Stricker 28 – 9
relaxations: chess 169; circus 201
religious conviction 202

school days 7 – 8
Senior Health Council, q.v.
Son, *see* Wagner-Jauregg, Theodor
Stepdaughter, devotion to 196, 197
university education 10 – 21
Venia legendi: neurology 36, 109, psychiatry 38
Vienna Medical Society
    at meetings 2, 66, 179
    lectures to 139, 153 – 4, 182
    use of libary 34, 46
Wagner-Jauregg, Karoline, née Schurz (1834 – 1915) (W-J's step-mother) 8
Wagner-Jauregg, Theodor (1903 – 92) (W-J's son) 3, 173, 196 – 7, 200
    on his father 2, 3
Wagner-Jauregg Oberösterreichische Landes-Nervenklinik 203
war neuroses 103 – 7
Wassermann, August von (1866 – 1925) 157
Wassermann test 157, 164, 166, 171, 173
Weber, Sonya, née Escherich 50
Weichbrodt, Raphael (b. 1886) 161
Weinheber, Josef (1892 – 1945) 179
Weitlof, Dr. 51, 61
Wernicke, Carl (1848 – 1905) 50
Wethmar, R. 170
Whittingham Mental Hospital, Liverpool 208
Wiesel, Josef (b. 1876) 140
women: admission to medical study at Vienna University 76
writing defects: improved by malaria therapy 164
Wundt, Wilhelm (1832 – 1920) 107

X-rays in treatment of GPI 173

Yorke, Warrington (1883 – 1943) 208

Zakon, S.J. 154, 155
Zuckerkandl, Emil (1849 – 1910) 76, 85, 86

*For W-J's researches and writings *see* the entries in the body of the Index and the references at the end of Chapters 1 – 4 and 6 – 11. Two lists of W-J's scientific writings were published in *Wien. Med. Wschr*, 1928, 78: 892 – 4 and 1937, 87: 254 – 5.